JOIN SO MANY OTHERS WHO DECIDED TO DO THE 7 DAY JUMP START AND GOT RESULTS.

ARE YOU NEXT?

"Your programs pushed me past my comfort zones. I'm finished with the program but I have learned things that I will continue doing to make a stronger healthier ME! I love the strength I have! I have new fit goals I'm working towards now, but thanks to your program and method of training I KNOW it's possible and I feel armed with the info I need!" —STACEY

"When it came to eating, I didn't know what I was doing: I'd count calories, eat clean for a week and go on a food splurge over the weekends. I wasn't happy, always disappointed at myself, I just didn't have self-control at all. The 7 Day Jump Start was easy to follow, and it totally changed my life!" —BULELWA

"I've just started a new job with a lot of night shifts and driving. I started the 7 Day Jump Start again and have been following steadily. I went from 164 lbs to 149 lbs in about 3 weeks. I can feel all my clothes are loose and I can definitely see the difference! I wanted Natalie to know that her program works—it truly does!" —TANYA

"Thank you so much for giving me back my life; not only for me but for my 2-year-old daughter and my husband. I have lost pounds and have gone from a size 10 to a size 4! I am so grateful for the encouragement that you post on your Instagram and Facebook to keep me going when I'm down. I have been motivated to pass on your gift you have given me!" —SHARLYN

"Hey Natalie. I wanted to say thank you for all your help. I purchased a few of your recipe books and it really helped me shed a lot of weight, not to mention your exercise plans. I've changed my lifestyle to a fit one, thanks to you as an inspiration. Thank you so much for your guidance and your delicious recipes." —FRANK

"The program was a game changer! I, too, have an autoimmune issue with Vitiligo, and after reading the materials and doing some research, I realized there were people who had slowed and even reversed the effects by eliminating gluten and wheat from their diet. The plan was so easy because I didn't have to think about what to do, I could just do it. The shopping list and even when to eat were all right there. I lost 10 pounds during 4 weeks." —KUNYA

"Wow! Where do I begin? The program literally changed my life. Your recipes were delicious, the exercises were fun, and your words were inspiring. When I felt like slacking off you gave me the motivation to keep on following this journey and reminded me of why I started it in the first place." —ROSE

"I've been following you for a few years and you've been so helpful. I've tried so many ways to lose weight and I've been the most successful with your guidelines (I started off with the 7 Day Jump Start). I lost 20 pounds gradually on my own and the last 20–25 with your program. It was not a diet, or a quick fix, but it was a lifestyle change which is realistic!!" —ELIF

 "I've lost 40 pounds and am soooo happy :). To maintain, I currently do my own body weight exercises at home and regularly follow Natalie's updates/tutorials videos that she uploads with different body weight exercises, as well as following a healthy unprocessed diet." —VEENA

Natalie Jill's

7 DAY JUMP START

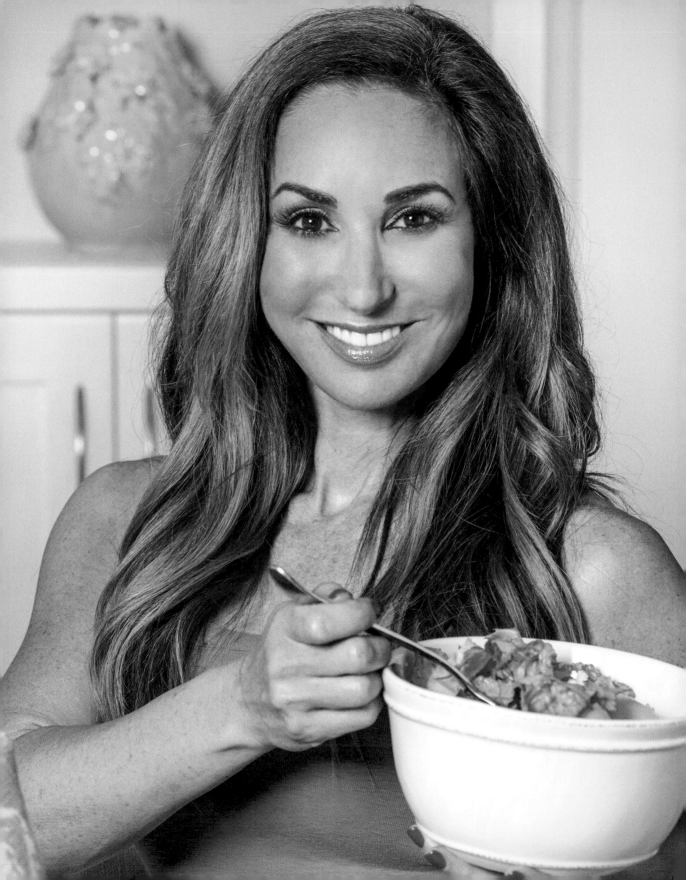

Natalie Jill's

7 DAY
JUMP
START

WITH SUPER EASY RECIPES

UNPROCESS
YOUR DIET

Lose up to 5–7 Pounds the First Week

Da Capo

LIFE
LONG

A MEMBER OF THE PERSEUS BOOKS GROUP

Copyright © 2016 by 212 Marketing Video Production, Inc.
Photos credits:
Food images and some of the commercial images by Mandy Schaffer.
Exercise images and some of the commercial images by Natalie Minh

Set in 11-point Adobe Caslon Pro

Library of Congress Control Number: 2016932032

First Da Capo Press edition 2016
Hardcover ISBN: 978-0-7382-1912-7
Ebook ISBN: 978-0-7382-1913-4

Published by Da Capo Press
A Member of the Perseus Books Group
www.dacapopress.com

Note: The information in this book is true and complete to the best of our knowledge. This book is intended only as an informative guide for those wishing to know more about health issues. In no way is this book intended to replace, countermand, or conflict with the advice given to you by your own physician. The ultimate decision concerning care should be made between you and your doctor. We strongly recommend you follow his or her advice. Information in this book is general and is offered with no guarantees on the part of the authors or Da Capo Press. The authors and publisher disclaim all liability in connection with the use of this book.

Da Capo Press books are available at special discounts for bulk purchases in the U.S. by corporations, institutions, and other organizations. For more information, please contact the Special Markets Department at the Perseus Books Group, 2300 Chestnut Street, Suite 200, Philadelphia, PA, 19103, or call (800) 810-4145, ext. 5000, or e-mail special.markets@perseusbooks.com.

10 9 8 7 6 5 4 3 2

To my dad—You left this earth way too young. If you had eaten more meals like the ones in this book, maybe you would still be here today to enjoy life with me. I miss and love you always.

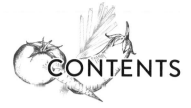

CONTENTS

PART 2: THE RECIPES

PART 3: FIT, HEALTHY, AND HAPPY . . . FOR LIFE!

Natalie Jill's

7 DAY JUMP START

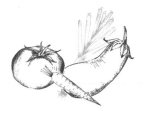

INTRODUCTION

NOT too many years ago, I was a new mom, more than sixty pounds heavier than I am today. I was working sixty hours a week, yet struggling financially because I was going through a divorce during an economic downturn. Worst of all, everything "bad" was happening at once, and I was completely overwhelmed. I was at rock bottom: depressed, confused, and feeling out of control with no idea how to find my way out.

Several years before everything came crashing down around me, I had been diagnosed with celiac disease. This was way before it was well known, and there were no "gluten-free" labels on products. When I first started eating gluten-free years ago, I relied on planning, as I had to eat naturally unprocessed foods to avoid gluten. As the years went by, more and more gluten-free packaged foods were coming onto the market. During this

busy and stressful time of my life, I got away from eating natural foods, and I turned to the convenient, but highly processed gluten-free foods. They sure tasted great, but I had a feeling that the "new" gluten-free pizzas, muffins, and breads were the culprits behind my weight gain.

When everything feels like it is spiraling out of control, you have to start by taking control of ONE thing and working up from there. One of the easiest things to control is what you put into your body. If you do it right, it will pay huge dividends, as you will not only feel better, but you will have the energy to tackle your other problems. If I wanted to get my health and life back on track, I knew I had to unprocess my diet again. But it had to be done in such a way that would fit me and my busy lifestyle, while not missing the processed foods.

I researched for a while, but when I didn't find anyone else offering a simple, easy-to-follow approach to unprocessed eating, I decided to create one myself.

You know what? It worked. I lost all the extra weight. I had forgotten how good I could feel, and my whole life began to change—for the better! Now, in my mid-forties, I'm in the best shape of my life and feel healthier than I did two decades ago! Going unprocessed resulted in the weight leaving and staying off, my mindset changing, my body looking and feeling younger, and ultimately, my becoming truly happy. As a bonus, I found my true calling: helping others to become the best version of themselves. I did this mostly through social media, where I serve as a fitness, nutrition, and motivational mentor to millions of people across the globe.

Celiac disease—a painful and fatiguing illness in which a person is unable to digest gluten—ended up becoming the best thing that could have happened to me, because ditching gluten was the first step toward unprocessing my diet. It turns out that you can lose weight and look and feel fantastic by dropping processed foods. I've figured out a way to make it easy, delicious, and fun, as my many followers who have lost the weight and changed their lives through the 7 Day Jump Start can attest to.

This book combines my best rules, recipes, and tools for eating an unprocessed naturally gluten-free diet. Most readers with 15 or more pounds to lose will typically lose up to 5 to 7 pounds in the first week, then lose, on average, about 2 pounds each week that follows, and achieve their total weight-loss goals in a matter of weeks or months—by making the 7 Day Jump Start their new lifestyle. Making it a lifestyle is important, as this is basically how I have eaten for many years now.

In these pages, I'll address every question, concern, need, and solution you might confront when unprocessing your life for the first time, or the umpteenth time for those of you who have yo-yoed back and forth for years. Don't worry. I've made it easy to follow, and you won't find it confusing or complex at all. In addition to my favorite new recipes, I'll share with you practical meal plans, guidelines, and life-changing tips about energy, hunger, and cravings, in addition to inspirational stories from other people just like you, who have successfully unprocessed their nutrition, and their lives.

When you harness the life-changing power of my 7 Day Jump Start, you'll tackle the hardest step of eating healthy, and you'll feel better than you have in years. You might even decide to start fitness modeling at the age of thirty-nine like I did. But even if you don't, you can still look like you could!

In a market of extreme and restrictive programs, my approach is accessible and fun. Plus, it takes just seven short days to get results and get going. You can do anything for seven days, especially when you see the power it has to truly change your life in such a short period of time. Let me show you how!

PART 1

THE

PROGRAM

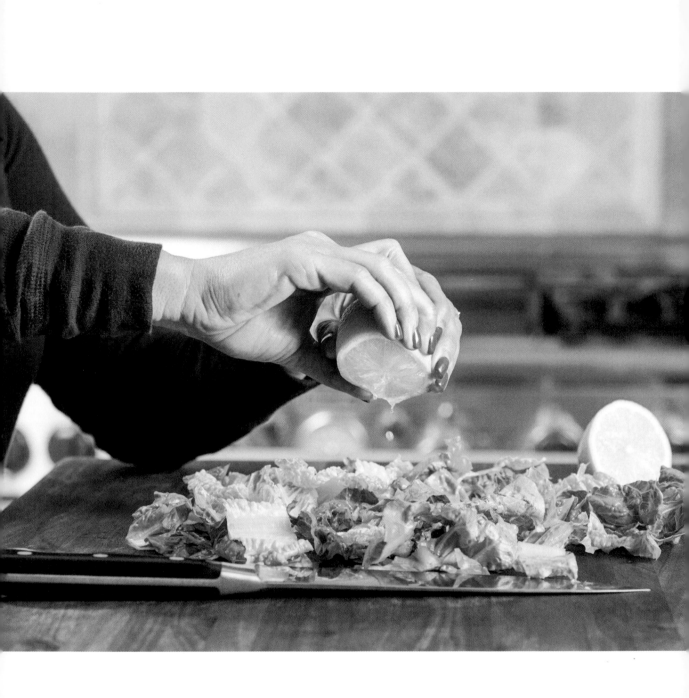

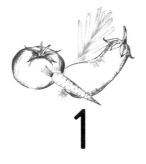

1

ROCK BOTTOM IS A SPRINGBOARD TO SUCCESS!

"Excuses or solutions . . . YOU decide!"

A little more than fifteen years ago, I experienced horrible abdominal pain every time I ate. Although I exercised somewhat regularly and I appeared to be a healthy, fit, and energetic person, I was struggling. On good days, it was a mild stomachache, but more often it was painful bloating and intense cramping accompanied by excessive fatigue. What no one knew at that time, including me, was that my immune system was attacking my own body. I was seriously ill and getting worse every day.

My illness started with the types of symptoms that you try to ignore. I experienced excessive tiredness in the afternoons, extreme hunger all the time but bloated every time I ate, with intense stomach cramping after each meal.

I quietly tried to self-diagnose and self-medicate. I was drinking a bottle of Mylanta a day to deal with the cramping, swallowing Beano before meals to try to deter the bloating, and I drank caffeine every afternoon to stay awake. I had been eating a lot of antioxidant-rich foods, so I thought that maybe I had been eating too many vegetables, too much fiber. I rationalized that white flour products were supposed to be good for stomachaches, so I reduced my veggies and fruit, adding more pasta, bread, and other bland starches to my diet. Things only got worse.

In addition to the other symptoms, a strange pain would develop in my chest after every meal. I had read several articles about fatigue and heart disease. As my dad had died very young of a sudden heart attack, I started worrying that maybe it was my heart. I consulted with my internist, made an appointment with a cardiologist, and even went to the emergency room.

After all of these visits, they told me that what I was experiencing was normal and they all made me feel like a hypochondriac. I did begin to feel like this was really all just in my head. I mean, all of the experts said, and their tests confirmed, that I was fine. It took a toll on me, and a mild depression set in.

By this time, my lower abdominal pain intensified, and I thought maybe my OB-GYN could help me. When she saw me, she told me I might have polycystic ovaries and gave me birth control pills to help the pain. I thought I had my solution, but the pain continued.

As the weeks and months went by, my condition continued to worsen. My lymph nodes started acting up, and I would get pea-size lumps in my neck, my groin, and my underarms. Did I have cancer? What was wrong with me? I was getting scared and knew something was really wrong. As I had been focused on health and fitness from an early age after losing my dad, I knew I had to take control of the situation and find solutions!

I went back to the internist and, almost embarrassed, made him listen to all of my symptoms again. He still didn't have a clue what my problem was, but because I mentioned that the chest pain normally would happen after eating, he did recommend that I go see a gastroenterologist. After ten minutes, the GI doctor told me it was heartburn and prescribed a drug as the solution. When that didn't work, he gave me another drug. My stomach and chest pain continued to get worse, not better. I began losing interest in eating because, to me, eating was associated with pain. After several weeks, I stopped taking the medicine.

I went back to the doctor, who now told me it was stress. Relax, I was told. Well, maybe it was stress. Maybe I was making myself sick. So, I took yoga, I meditated, and I was committed to relaxing, but there was still no change in my symptoms.

There were more doctor visits; was it depression? An ulcer? An endoscope examination and a stomach biopsy showed no ulcer. I was diagnosed with IBS as well as "low pain tolerance." Would this explain why my chest hurt? That still didn't sound right to me, and these diagnoses added to the list from the previous two years—everything from chronic fatigue syndrome to polycystic ovaries, IBS, stress, depression. I decided I was done going to the doctor. Nothing was really wrong with me. It must all be in my head.

Then, two weeks after the endoscopy and biopsy, I received a phone call from a nurse. The biopsy showed signs of celiac disease. I had never heard of it. I looked it up online that night. I could not believe what I read—I was a textbook case for celiac disease! In a nutshell, a healthy stomach has little "fingers" called villi in it. In my stomach, it was almost as smooth as a bowling ball. Because I had celiac disease, the villi in my stomach were gone, and *that* was what was causing so many issues!

One of the hallmarks of celiac disease is that it is commonly misdiagnosed. What surprised me even more is that not one doctor I had been to had even suggested this as a possibility! I was *accidentally* diagnosed with celiac disease. They weren't even looking for it.

To make matters even more ridiculous, celiac disease is an autoimmune disease, and the tendency toward acquiring an autoimmune disease is genetic. Since many of my family members suffer from other autoimmune diseases, I wondered, how did all of these doctors miss this? It is because celiac disease was still not widely known or understood.

After my celiac diagnosis, my doctor's advice sounded easy at first: "Just look for foods without gluten as an ingredient." Turns out that was a lot harder than I thought. When you think back to the late 1990s, nobody knew what "gluten-free" was all about. There were no gluten-free sections at grocery stores or gluten-free labels on foods. I knew that gluten was the protein found in wheat, barley, and rye, but I had no idea how many foods contained those ingredients. Obviously bread, pasta, and crackers were off the menu. But gluten works its way into all sorts of processed foods, including candy, preservatives, marinades, soy sauce, and deli meats, as well as many fillers and thickening agents.

For this reason, it can be hard to spot all the different names for gluten. I found that the absolute surefire, easiest way to avoid gluten was simply to eat real, unprocessed food! Yes, it was *that* simple!

I thought that I ate pretty healthy before, but now I would be taking it up a notch and to truly eat healthy, as doing so was crucial to *feeling* healthy and pain-free. At first, I missed the foods I used to eat, but after just a few days of being gluten-free, it was no longer a concern, because every single symptom went away! I had forgotten how good feeling "normal" could be. And once I was feeling better, my whole life was different. I had renewed confidence, and I was excited to tackle each day. My relationships felt more like a blessing than a burden. It was amazing to know that I could be completely free of pain just by eating a certain way.

MY ROCK BOTTOM: SAYING GOOD-BYE TO MY DREAM LIFE

Several years after my celiac diagnosis, I was having a tough time. Not just any tough time, but one of those rock bottom times when everything that can go wrong, does.

It started when I was just about to have my daughter. Anyone who looked at me from the outside would have thought I had the perfect life. I had the nice house, nice car, nice job, nice husband, and I lived in San Diego with its nice weather. But all of that was just a facade. On the inside, I was miserable and things were spiraling out of control.

At the time, I was working sixty-plus hours a week as a national sales manager for a medical device company and was traveling weekly. I was on the road three to five days every week, and had been for years. I remember sitting at home on what should have been a relaxing Sunday afternoon, but instead I was thinking that I had to be up super early to get to the airport on time. Monday was almost here, and I was about to get on an airplane *again*. The last thing I felt like doing while eight months pregnant was travel cross-country on a six a.m. flight the next morning.

In addition to that, I was married to someone whom had been my best friend and who I did everything with, but those days had somehow disappeared and my marriage was falling apart. It didn't help that my closest girlfriends and my family all lived three thousand miles away on the East Coast and I was out in California.

I had already gained 50 pounds on my 5′2″ frame and still had a month of pregnancy to go. I was living in a house I couldn't afford with somebody I no longer felt connected to; I didn't know how I was going to pay the bills or how I was going to escape the situation I had somehow gotten myself into. I was stressing about maternity leave and how my financial problems would likely get worse once I wasn't able to travel each week. I probably would have to take a voluntary demotion to a position with less travel if I wanted to be there for my daughter. I was feeling lonely and afraid, and everything seemed so out of control. I hated what my life had become.

Not only had I always been a positive, upbeat, happy person, but I had always been so excited about having a daughter. Now my greatest wish was coming true and everything else was falling apart all around me. I had never felt like this before in my entire life.

After my daughter was born, matters spiraled further out of control. I took that voluntary demotion at work so I could be home to raise my daughter. That meant I could no longer afford my dream home anymore, and the real estate crash had simultaneously wiped out my equity, something I had invested my hard-earned money in.

One day when I stopped to get gas on my way back from work, I got out of my car like I always did, slid in my credit card, and . . . *declined*. Never in my life had I had a credit card decline. I called the credit card company to see what the error was. Sure enough, they had cut me off. Even though I had never missed or been late on a payment to them, they canceled my cards because of the debt from my house.

I sat there in the passenger seat with the gas pump attached to my car, but I had no money to put in it. There I was, a grown woman who had always taken care of herself, calling my mom, bawling my eyes out because I couldn't even put gas in my car. As somebody who had always prided herself on being financially responsible, I couldn't believe this was happening to me. After all, my dad was an accountant, and if I had learned anything from him, it was how to properly manage money.

My mom ended up wiring me money and co-signing on a new credit card so that I could at least have a working credit card. I went home and had an ugly cry. Yes, the ugly cry. The kind you do alone and that you hope nobody hears or sees. Where you ponder whatever mess you got yourself into and feel sorry for yourself.

With my credit cards being canceled and the stock market in free fall, the financially sound life I had built over many years was gone. My husband and I filed for divorce. I had to share custody of my daughter, which meant less time with the one person who meant the world to me. I was overweight, depressed, and more alone than I had ever been in my life, and I was only thirty-six. Everything I had been years before—confident, successful, positive, energetic, and happy—was gone. I didn't know who that girl was anymore. The dream life and outside appearance I had worked so hard for had come to an end.

I was still eating gluten-free, but I was about 60 pounds heavier than I am today and suffering from depression, hunger, grumpiness, and hormone fluctuations. What had changed? I was miserable and ate terribly. I used food to comfort me. As much as I hate to admit it, trips to the drive-through for French fries and fudge sundaes became a regular part of my diet while I was pregnant. Things were so bad, it was like I lost a part of myself. So sad to think that my happiness came from two fast food items.

Not only was the fast food not helping, but due to increased public awareness about gluten intolerance, a whole industry of processed gluten-free foods had sprung up over the past several years. Convenience foods that were once off the table for somebody with celiac disease were again an option for me. It became very easy to rely on the gluten-free packaged foods that were now available at every grocery store. From gluten-free breads to gluten-free pizza and pasta, nothing seemed to be off-limits anymore.

So much for eating "real food" like I had when I was diagnosed with celiac disease. Processed gluten-free foods were convenient, they gave me short-term happiness, and they kept my celiac symptoms in check. But they sure weren't doing my body any favors. I had a suspicion the gluten-free cookies, muffins, and pizzas might have something to do with my weight gain, but for a period of time there, I was too busy having a pity party to care.

The lowest point of this rock bottom moment in my life was catching a glimpse of myself walking past the mirrored windows of a shopping center while I was pushing the stroller and walking my dogs, Bean and Cali. That was the final straw. I saw stuff hanging in places it never had before. I felt disgusting. I didn't recognize myself. I had heard from so many women that once you have a baby, you just can't get your body back, that you will always have the baby weight. But what I had gained was a lot more than just normal baby weight. That was not what I wanted for myself.

After some serious soul searching, I decided that doing nothing and continuing down this path was a guaranteed dead-end decision. It can be tough to really look at your life and take responsibility for things that might not have gone as planned, but that's what I had to do. I aspired to be the person I once was and possibly even better. I was determined not to give up! I had to take personal responsibility for my situation, my life, and my future. I did not wallow in my excuses. I finally asked myself: "What is the opportunity in all of this?"

UNPROCESSING MY DIET AND CREATING A HEALTHY LIFESTYLE

It took some time, but I finally picked myself up. I thought back to when I was a sales director, and how I taught all the sales reps about setting goals and creating a vision to achieve them. The thing is, since my life had been pretty good, I never actually did the work myself. Now was the time for me to take action and take the steps I had helped so many others take. I had to get my life and my health back on track. I would finally do all the things I had been telling others to do for years. Yes, it took some effort, but it felt good to "do" instead of just to "teach," if you know what I mean.

I knew that nutrition was key, so rather than continuing with a diet of gluten-free versions of bread, pasta, and other processed foods, I would give up gluten the way I had in the first place, by unprocessing my diet and my lifestyle. I knew that unprocessing my diet needed to be as simple, straightforward,

delicious, and fun as those packaged gluten-free muffins and frozen pizzas. But when I looked to find books or other information on giving up packaged food or eating a clean diet, they were all about intensive overhauls that were too extreme and restrictive to fit into my busy life.

I knew that anything too restrictive couldn't be sustained for the long haul, and I was in it for the long haul. From fat-free, sugar-free, low- and no-carb diets, to vegetarianism and veganism, I found their all-consuming approaches to clean eating overwhelming and intimidating. I figured most people were probably like me and had no interest in strict elimination diets that relied more on willpower than anything else, as they removed entire food groups or restricted certain nutrients, or in juice cleanses that practically meant giving up eating altogether! I wanted something simple that I could read and understand quickly. When I couldn't find it, I decided to start putting something together for myself. As part of my transformation, I worked with these questions:

- What would happen if everyone gave themselves a chance to eat the right way?
- What if eating an unprocessed diet for a week was made easy and delicious for even the busiest of people?
- And what if you only had to commit to an unprocessed lifestyle for seven days to drop up to five pounds and jump start your weight loss?

Could it be fun? Could it be a life-changer? It sure was!

MAPPING OUT MY GOALS: BECOME A FITNESS MODEL AT AGE THIRTY-NINE?

Doing what I had taught others in corporate America to do for years, I first made a vision board to map out my goals and put my plan into place (read more about vision boards on page 24). I pulled out fit-looking people and fitness models, because I knew deep down that I could be a fit person again. I pulled out happy couples, I pulled out pictures of money, and I pulled out an ocean view. I put the words *fitness model* on the board.

Why? Because it was so far from how I was feeling. I was out of shape, but I knew deep down that this was possible. You have to get your mind believing in something if you have any hope of ever achieving it. I knew that getting my mind right would be the first step. If I could get my mind right and get that negative voice in my head in check, I could work my way out of this hole. I started looking at my vision board every night. I thought that if I could just move one step toward what I saw on it every day, maybe I could get somewhere.

I started telling my friends that I was going to become a fitness model. Most everyone laughed and told me I could never be a fitness model, especially starting at age thirty-nine. I didn't let that discourage me. In fact, I told them I was going to be on the cover of three fitness magazines. At that point I didn't really care what people thought. I had hit rock bottom. There was nowhere to go but up.

As time went on, I shared what I was doing on Facebook. I found people who would believe in me and support me along the way. As I was working out and getting in shape, I started sharing my story and posting what I was eating. I was surprised to find out how many people were hungry for easy-to-understand instructions and recipes to unprocess their diets and lives one step at a time. I had no idea that things would end up where they are today, with a huge social media following including well over a million followers just on Facebook. People were sharing the information I put out there, and it was genuinely helping them.

From my first posts, people would ask how I made my recipes, and next thing you know they were asking if I had a recipe book. So I gathered photos that I took with my BlackBerry (does anyone still have a Black-Berry?!), created my own website, and started selling my recipe book from the site.

People began asking for more. They loved the recipes, but they wanted to know how I ate each day and how to use those recipes. So I took some time and created what's now called the 7 Day Jump Start—"The Plan." It became a huge hit, not because it was a beautiful book or I had a big marketing plan, but because I just kept sharing and helping others while moving in the direction of success.

AN EARLY WAKE-UP CALL

WHILE my celiac diagnosis was a big catalyst in terms of taking charge of my health and unprocessing my diet, my interest in fitness and nutrition actually started in my early twenties.

I was twenty-one, finishing college, waiting tables for work, and getting ready to backpack through Europe for a month. I was young, happy, carefree, and excited about life. I wasn't thinking about a future with family, kids, and a career down the road, and I certainly didn't think about a future without my dad. My dad was my world, and I admired him greatly. He thought I was a "health nut" compared to him, and would tease me about my exercise and eating habits.

Everything changed the evening of July 2, 1994. It was a busy day at work, and I received a call from the office phone. All I heard was "Dad's in the hospital . . ." I grabbed my stuff and off I went. By the time I got to the hospital, he was already gone.

No "he had a heart attack, now let's change habits." No warnings. Just *boom*! Gone. Done. No hugs. No good-byes. No last words. It was not an underlying genetic disease that got him. Like so many, his death was entirely preventable, as it was a direct result of poor nutrition and lack of physical activity. He was only forty-nine. I was twenty-two, my brother was twenty, and my sister was only twelve. He left us without a dad, and he left my young mom a widow.

I miss him so much, and at the same time, I am angry that he wouldn't listen. Angry that he didn't think it was important to change his lifestyle so he could be with us today to watch his kids become adults and raise their own children.

I post "A Letter to Dad" on social media each year on the anniversary of his passing (www.nataliejillfitness.com/letter-to-dad/). One thing is consistent—the number of people who respond with stories of losing somebody they cared about way too early because the person didn't take their health in their own hands before it was too late. I share this story to stress how important it is to follow a healthy lifestyle, not just for *you* but for your loved ones, too!

It really hit me how crucial it was to take good care of myself. I needed to maintain more awareness of my health, because I didn't want to go down the same road my father had taken. As I look back, it's clear that his death was the initial catalyst that started me down the path I am on today.

So please, stop the excuses for any habits that are self-inflicting, life-threatening diseases. The formula is not that difficult: eat clean, natural, unprocessed foods, and just move. Walk, walk, and walk some more. Be active. Don't let a sedentary life become you. Remember that your decisions affect the lives of more people than just yourself, people who want you around for a long time, including people who might not even be born yet, like kids and grandkids. My daughter, Penelope, has three of her four grandparents, and always asks, "Where is grandpa, when is he coming?" or, "What happened to grandpa?"

I ultimately created my fitness and nutrition plans to make it easy for others so they could learn from my loss instead of having to experience it themselves. I want you to benefit from my wake-up call. Embrace a healthy lifestyle of proper eating and fitness habits, and the odds are on your side that you will live a happier, healthier, and longer life.

MAKING MY OWN LUCK: THE BIRTH OF THE 7 DAY JUMP START

All that plugging away and persistence paid off. I made my own luck! At thirty-nine I *did* become a fitness model, and I became a fitness, nutrition, and motivational mentor to so many people. I ended up on the covers of *more than* three magazines and built a thriving fitness business from a place where no one believed in me. Now in my mid-forties, I am in the best shape of my life and feel better than I did in my twenties. Once I had control of my nutrition, I got the healthy body I was after, and things became clear. I turned my problems into opportunities and found solutions that worked! Once I did this, everything else fell into place. All this came from my rock bottom place, which, as it turns out, is a great place to rebuild. As crazy as it sounds, when things are really bad, there truly is only one place to go . . . and that is up!

> **"I decided I could reinvent my life. I listed out my goals and started to act as if I already was the person I wanted to become. And it worked!"**

Fast-forward a few short years, and I have literally millions of people who have been enjoying my fitness videos and lifestyle nutrition plans. Many of them have shared their weight-loss success stories and testimonials

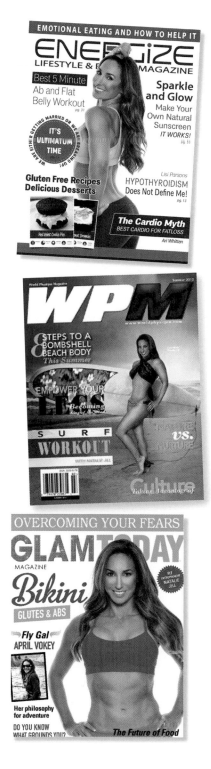

about reclaiming their lives, their identities, and their relationships by unprocessing their diets and everything else that comes along with it—you'll meet some of them and read their amazing stories here. When people have more energy and are in shape, they look and feel better, and this has a positive impact on every part of their lives.

Since the beginning, one thing that a lot of people consistently asked for is more recipes—specifically, more delicious unprocessed recipes to help them to jump start their weight loss and create a foundation for a new, healthy way of eating for a lifetime. And they wanted it in a book—so that's just what this book is all about! I can't wait for you to try all my new favorites—from blueberry almond muffins for breakfast to eggplant lasagna for dinner and strawberry chocolate cobbler for dessert. Are you in?

WHAT IS CELIAC DISEASE?

A PERSON who has celiac disease has a body that does not recognize gluten and does not digest it. Every time a person with celiac disease eats something containing gluten, their immune system attacks their digestive tract (specifically the small intestine), which can significantly interfere with the body's ability to absorb certain essential nutrients. Celiac disease can affect men and women across all ages and ethnic backgrounds.

A 100 percent gluten-free diet (completely avoiding wheat, barley, and rye) is the only existing treatment for celiac today. There are no pharmaceutical cures for celiac disease.

Approximately 1 in 133 Americans, or about 1 percent of the population, has celiac disease. A surprising fact I discovered is that it is estimated that 83 percent of Americans who have celiac disease are undiagnosed or wrongly diagnosed with other conditions. (I was far from being alone!) The average time a person waits to be correctly diagnosed is six to ten years. But with growing awareness of the disease, this is quickly changing.

If you have any of the combination of symptoms I had, talk to your doctor to find out if you should be tested. A blood test identifies the gene and a biopsy determines the extent of the damage. Untreated celiac disease can be very serious; it can lead to a number of other disorders including infertility, reduced bone density, neurological disorders, some cancers, and other autoimmune diseases. Treating celiac disease may alleviate all of your symptoms and can greatly lower your risk of digestive tract cancers. Plus, treating celiac disease by unprocessing your diet will make you healthier than you ever thought possible!

JOAN'S TRANSFORMATION:

From Diet Soda Addiction and Depression to Losing the Weight for Good

JOAN BEFORE

JOAN AFTER

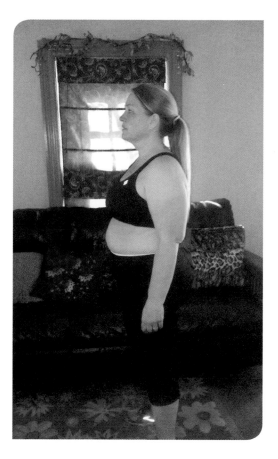

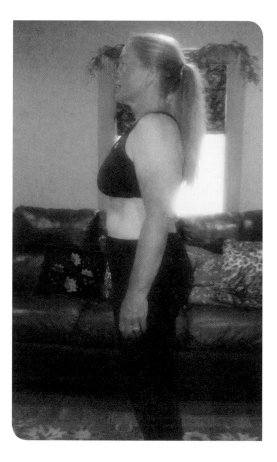

When everything changed for the worse: My family is very athletic, and we would take pride in it. I used to run every day and lifted weights for years. Then, around three years ago, I started working at the busiest restaurant in Providence, mainly at night. I took the job so I could be home more with the family and be more involved with the boys' school activities. I started developing some seriously bad eating habits: I would bring home cheesecake and an entree late at night and sit in front of the computer to unwind. I'd eat half of whatever I brought home, then make an ice cream cone. I'd drink four or five cans of Diet Mountain Dew a day—I drank Diet Mountain Dew for twenty-three years!

I no longer recognized myself: At my worst, I was 225 pounds, depressed, and totally miserable. I had to pack away nine bins of beautiful clothes that I no longer could fit into. My work pants were a size 40 waist. Never in my wildest nightmare did I ever think I would be this big. I had to buy a size 22 bathing suit. We live in the ocean state, and going to the beach is a favorite thing for us to do, but for the first time last summer, I was embarrassed to walk to the water.

Looking for a quick fix: I would try any diet that was new, and I tried diet pills. I was so desperate for the quick fix that when I heard that a well-known antidepressant helped one to lose weight, I went to the doctor and pretended I had most of the symptoms. Yes, I was depressed, but it was nothing a pill could help. I was so desperate that I called about LAP-BAND surgery, but wasn't qualified because I had to be 100 pounds overweight. I thought very seriously about trying to get to that point just so I could get the surgery.

Finding Natalie Jill: When I found Natalie Jill on Facebook, I subscribed, and kept reading and re-reading the testimonials. It took me another two months to try the 7 Day Jump Start, but *wow*, it was the best thing I have ever done for myself.

Making the change: When I committed to the 7 Day Jump Start, the first thing I had to do was quit drinking Diet Mountain Dew. In fact, I stopped all artificial sweeteners. The third day into my withdrawal from diet soda, my bones started to ache and I was so exhausted. I couldn't get comfortable and I couldn't even keep my eyes open that afternoon. It's hard to describe how horrible I actually felt. It was the worst experience in my entire life.

Feeling like a new person: The fourth day I felt like a whole new person. I was forty-nine years old and relearning how to eat. I was still heavy, of course, but there was a new energy about me. I went out and bought every single thing on Natalie's shopping list and followed the program to a T. I had really never eaten properly, and I wanted to make sure I didn't mess it up. And it is working! Yes, there are hard days when I am craving something sweet. I was worried about the traditional stop to the ice cream shop on the way back from the beach, but the protein shakes made with frozen fruit are an amazing alternative to ice cream. They taste like milk shakes, and I have my whole family hooked!

I started walking my dog for forty-five minutes every day, I've been taking aqua classes at the gym, and sometimes I'll swim laps with my husband. I am happy to say my relationship with my husband is just like it was years ago. My kids see such a huge difference in me, not only physically, but in my demeanor toward everything I do. I still volunteer my time to both elementary and middle schools, but I take care of me first. Honestly, I have not been this happy in many years.

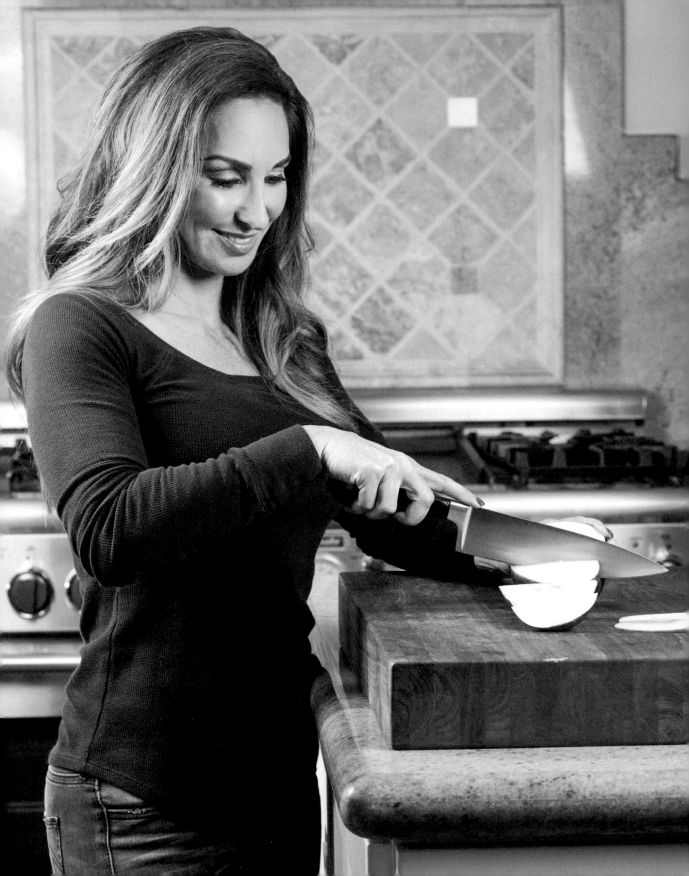

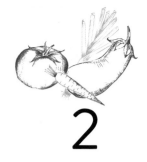

2

GETTING SET FOR YOUR 7 DAY JUMP START: *DECIDING* COMES FIRST

"Every step forward is a step in the right direction."

YOU'RE about to embark on a terrific journey, one that will not only change your diet and your weight, but also your life. I know what's possible for you because I know how it happened for me and for millions of my followers. You'll get into a good place mentally and emotionally. You'll take responsibility for your health and well-being, and find solutions rather than excuses. Whether you're merely trying to tighten up for swimsuit season, a special occasion, or you have never felt good about your weight your entire life, this plan will walk you through a proven system that will give you

the fundamentals not just for weight loss, but for overall success.

But first, did you know that how we *think* goes a long way toward our success? After working with thousands of people, I have come to find that success is dependent on a lot more than just calories and food selection. Success depends on many variables, but if one key variable isn't right, then it is next to impossible to reach your goals.

That one key is your mindset. In my programs, I have applied my twenty years of corporate goal achievement experience to helping you create a mindset for weight-loss success.

I learned how to harness the power of my mind—and you can too. I'm going to show you how I turned problems into opportunities.

After I had to give up my first home because I fell behind on the mortgage, if someone said, "It's too bad you lost your house," I'd respond, "It's awesome that I live in an affordable, cute house that I can walk to the beach from." When someone would comment, "It's too bad that you no longer have that high-powered sales job," I'd say, "It's awesome that I can spend my days working my own business and have the freedom to pick up my daughter from school." And when someone would say, "It's too bad you got divorced," I'd say, "I am so lucky to have found my soul mate at forty!" You can harness the power of your mind for health, weight loss—and anything else you want!

If you believe, you can achieve. Am I saying it's easy? Of course not. Am I saying that any reasonable thing you want is probably within your grasp? Yes, I am. I know you have challenges, perhaps very tough ones. I get that. My success didn't come easily—few accomplishments do. But I made up my mind that I would achieve my dreams. So can you.

Excuses or solutions? Everyone can make excuses, because each of us has challenges. In the end, it doesn't matter how big or small, how few or many. All that matters is how you choose to view those challenges. Do you consider your trials mere obstacles with potential solutions, or insurmountable, disabling difficulties?

Losing weight is so much more than what you eat or don't eat. That's a huge part, to be sure—but your most important weapon in the battle for weight control is your mind. You have to be consistent. It did not take a short period of time to get off track. It can't all be undone in a day, week, or month, no matter what the scale says. Be consistent, push through, commit to making things happen, and a new you will shine through. Take responsibility. Get to work. Your life depends on it.

> **"Commit to fit. Visualize it. Check excuses at the door. Make a plan. Carry it out. Encourage yourself, and get others on your team."**

When you get off track, instead of beating yourself up for all of the "bad things" you ate or did, list all of the good things you can *add* to your life: Can you add more positive friends, conversations, experiences? Add more, and make less room for the bad—adding, not subtracting, is a big part of this plan. Who's in?

> **"Decide that failure is not an option."**

WHAT KEEPS YOU MOTIVATED?

The 7 Day Jump Start is just that—a jump start. It's *not* the seven-day quick fix that you can try for a week and then go back to your

FINDING YOUR "WHY"

"I NEED to work out, but can't find the time . . ."

"I can't seem to stay (or get) motivated . . ."

"It's too hard to eat right . . ."

"I work out for a day or two, I don't see results, so I stop . . ."

Do any of these sound like you? If you are looking for answers why, I'm going to turn this back to you and ask a very important question: What is *your* why?

It is impossible to stay committed and determined to do anything unless you know your "why." The "why" is the real reason, the driving reason, that you want to change, work out, get healthy, or whatever it is that you truly want to do.

You can't change for someone else, and you can't change for superficial reasons. You can only change if your "why" becomes seriously important.

How do you find your "why"?

I'm going to help you do just that in a moment when I ask you to answer the questions in "What Keeps You Motivated?" I also want you to seriously consider making a vision board (see below) to reveal your deep desires and your "why."

I know some of you are thinking, "I don't need to do that." Well, let me tell you, all the successful people I've met make vision boards. Getting your mind right is so important, and a vision board is a great way to get started. Plus, you just might enjoy it! Take some time for *you,* do some soul-searching, and get serious in your thinking. Is it for your health? To feel great daily? For more energy? To be around and active for your children? There is no wrong "why"; it just needs to have meaning and be personal to *you.*

Once you get to the root of your "why," it changes and drives you. All of a sudden, solutions to your problems will start presenting themselves to you. The hurdles become crystal clear, and you start to take action and make things happen. All because you found out what drives you.

Discovering your "why" is the most important step to changing, as it gets your mind right. Once you find your "why" and your mind becomes focused, you can't be stopped! When you are ready to make changes and turn your life around, find your "why" and the solution will find its way to you.

---

old habits. Rather, it's the beginning of a lifestyle program designed to give you a solid nutritional base that will translate into long-term healthy eating habits.

You'll be taking these next seven days to learn the foods that are best for your body, and you will start to lose the bloat, lose the sluggishness, start to gain the energy, and start to drop the extra weight. It's a jump start to give you the foundation to change your life for the better. My hope is that by seeing the quick results, you'll be more likely to stick with this way of eating for the long term. The longer you stick with eating unprocessed foods, the more you'll see changes, create new habits, and build a whole new lifestyle and the foundation to lose the weight *and* keep it off for good!

Before we get to eat all that delicious food, before you grab your car keys (extra points for jumping on your bicycle or lacing up your walking shoes!) and head to the grocery store to stock up on healthy food for the next seven days, ask yourself this: *Why do you want to do this program?*

Let's go a little deeper—beyond dieting and achieving weight-loss goals—and think about what motivated you to embark on this 7 day journey. Why is this so important for you? I want to make sure you want to do it bad enough to not only stick through the seven days, but to keep the new habits going.

Take a break and stop thinking about the kids, family, work, deadlines, or whatever else is on your mind. It's time to get self-centered for a few minutes, because we are going to take some time to focus on your favorite person—you!

The beauty of this program is that it's designed to give you a framework to change your lifestyle so that you can get what you want out of life. If you outline your goals first, it will help you reach the finish line, because it will allow you to focus on what is *really* important to you, and not allow you to get sidetracked with any short-term "tests" that you will encounter. There will be times when you will want to dive spoon-first into a huge dessert, or stuff your face with _____ [insert favorite guilty pleasure here], but staying focused on why you want this in the long run will help curb your desire to cheat and keep you focused on your goals and what is important to you. Your goal can be completely different from those of your friends or anyone else's. That doesn't matter. What matters is that you get what *you* want. That's what separates this system from the rest. It's all about you!

I want you to start taking control of your future. How many times have you set out to do something but never started, much less completed the task? It's OK—you can admit it. Almost everybody has done this at one time or another. Millions of people have set out to read a book, lose weight, or learn a skill, but never ended up doing it because they didn't have a structure to keep them on track. I'm giving you that structure. I want you to start by answering the following five questions.

Now let's grab a pen and some paper. It's time to start writing:

1. What is important to you?

Don't worry—there are no right or wrong answers. Just write it out. What do you find most important? Your spouse? Your health? Your friends? Why do you want to be a healthier and thinner you?

2. What are your goals?

List out your fantasy, long-term, short-term, and daily goals. Be as detailed and free-thinking as possible without trying to monitor your thoughts. Here are some examples:

Fantasy goals: If I could have any life that I wanted, what would it look like? How would I feel? Would I feel fit and lean? Who would I be surrounded by? Where would I live? Who would I be friends with? How would I live? Where would I spend my time? What would my career be? What would my priorities be? Would I be happy?

Long-term goals: How do I see myself in the next five to ten years? What is my lifestyle? (Be as specific and detailed as possible. Examples: thin, fit, toned, pain-free, working out frequently, happy, in a new career, making more money.) How do you want to feel long-term? Take time to envision this.

Short-term goals: What needs to happen to get you to these long-term goals? What do I need to do this year? Where do I want to be a year from now? What can I control or change? What can I do this week to jump start my goals?

Daily goals: What do I need to do today and every day to achieve my goals? What time do I need to wake up each day? What foods do I need to prepare the night before? What days and times do I need to work out, shop for groceries, and so on? What friends do I need to let out of my life, and whom do I need to begin to surround myself with?

3. What is your main reason for wanting to lose weight and adopt a healthy lifestyle?

Is it so you can play with your kids or grandkids? Is it because you want to be able to walk up a flight of stairs without getting out of breath? Is it because you want to live longer? Is it because you have a lifelong dream of running a marathon? Do you just want your jeans to fit better?

Remember, there are no right or wrong answers; it's all about what is important to you.

4. Why is the reason stated above so important to you, and how will losing weight and changing your lifestyle impact your life?

Is it so you can be alive to see and experience your kids' lives and eventually their kids' lives? So you can be there to see them graduate or get married?

5. Who are the people in your life who will support you on your path toward a fit and healthy lifestyle?

Is it your partner, your children, your friends, coworkers, or a dedicated support group?

Keep the answers to these questions close to your bed. Review them before you go to sleep and first thing in the morning. The more you review why this is important to you, the easier it will be for you to accomplish your goals. As you continue to review your answers, you will see your mindset change. By working toward these goals, you can live your dreams. Your mind will move away from negativity and doubt and toward a more and more positive state. From there the rest will come easy. From there anything becomes possible!

"I could reinvent my life. I listed out my goals. I made a vision board and I decided to practice what I knew would work; to act as if I was already the person I wanted to become. I decided to do the work."

Remember, even with the best of intentions, self-motivation can fade quickly or die completely at the first bump in the road. That is why it is so important to have something bigger that you are working toward. When you have your sights set on something, it is next to impossible to get easily sidetracked. So now that you've found your motivation, continue to keep focused on your goals. One really effective way of defining your true goals and visions and to start moving forward in the direction of achieving them is by using a vision board.

IF YOU CAN VISUALIZE IT, YOU CAN ACHIEVE IT: CREATING A VISION BOARD

Who do you want to become? Do you want to be healthier? Stronger? Slimmer? Fitter?

Live in a new home? Do you want to drive a new car? Have a family? Have a great relationship?

If you can *visualize* those things happening, you can achieve them! I am not discounting the fact that you have to *work* for results. Believe me, you do. There are no shortcuts to the work, but without visualizing the process first, you won't ever get started. You can't just visualize, wish, and dream—you have to do the work. Creating a vision board is a very effective part of the goal-setting process; it's a powerful tool to help keep you on track while working on achieving your goals. I've gained so much from using vision boards over the years by identifying, clarifying, and focusing on specific life goals that I've wanted to accomplish.

Remember, transformation starts in the mind. You have to want it, believe it, and visualize it. If you can visualize your transformation—your goals, your desires—and continue to visualize them every day, everywhere, you will move toward them.

I made my first vision board when I was in a bad place. I was going through a divorce, I was a new mom, I was leaving a house I loved, and I was feeling sad and hopeless. I was just beginning to pick up the pieces and move on with a better life. I cut out magazine pictures of happy people and things that made me feel joy, and began busily gluing them onto a cardboard background. At the time, what I put on the board seemed impossible. They were all things I wanted and wished for but seemed so far out of reach. I included them on my vision board anyway and started to do the work toward achieving them. At the time I had no idea how important (or prophetic!) my vision board would become.

The crazy thing is when I look at that vision board now, I see that just about every single thing has come to fruition!

You don't need any special tools or artistic skills to make a vision board. All you need is a blank poster board, some roll-on glue, scissors, your favorite magazines, and a sense of adventure.

HOW TO MAKE A VISION BOARD

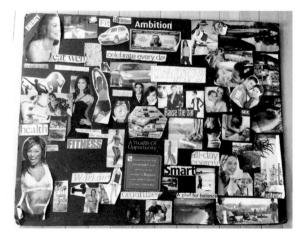

Step 1: Cut out/collect images and text that speak to you and represent your goals and what you want your life to look like. This isn't about immediately gravitating toward familiar pictures like expensive cars, skinny models, and designer clothes. Look to the unexpected. Look to the abstract. I want you to dig deep and use pictures that have a greater meaning for you. The more magazines you can go through, the better. Use housing, vacation, fitness, style, and business magazines. Start cutting and tearing. Cut out any picture, phrase, or word that appeals to you. Don't go into this with a plan or direction just see what appeals to you and make that pile!

Step 2: Get yourself a nice piece of poster board, a glue stick, and/or some tape, and have fun pasting your images into a collage. Don't stress about where each image goes; just let it come together naturally. This is for *you*, not your spouse or your children or your friends. Put images on the board that you like, and don't worry about what anyone else thinks. Remember, your images may say something completely different to someone else, so know that this is a deeply personal process.

Step 3: Keep your vision board where it can inspire you when you need it. The purpose of your vision board is to help you lead yourself to the future you desire. Don't feel the need to place it on display or explain yourself to others—I want the vision board to help fuel your internal dialogue along with your external actions. Just make sure to put your vision board somewhere that you will see it on a daily basis.

Amazing things happen once you create and use your vision board. You start to move toward your vision and you start to do the work to make your goals happen. I have made a vision board every year for the last several years, and it is always amazing to look back at previous vision boards—those visions more often than not have come to fruition. So what are you waiting for? Go create your own vision board!

I was in Palm Desert a little while back on a hike with my husband, Brooks, and one of his good friends. We were at a strenuous part of the hike—it was actually more like a rock climb at this point. His friend was above me and reached out to give me a helping hand. As I reached up to grab his hand, I had a déjà-vu moment. The exact picture of what was in front of me was on the vision board I had created a while back!

You've identified your goals, both short-term and long-term. You've created a vision board to map out your future success. You've set the stage for becoming the *you* you've always dreamed of. Congratulations! You've completed the crucial first step. Now it's time to dive into the 7 Day Jump Start.

In the chapters that follow, I'll teach you how to unprocess your diet (and you'll learn how delicious it can be!), give you an understanding of the importance of protein, fat, and carbs so you can learn how to build a perfectly balanced meal, and then I'll map out what you'll be eating and what you'll be avoiding for the next seven days and beyond. Then we'll jump into the kitchen and cook our way through the most delicious unprocessed dishes you can imagine!

JIM'S TRANSFORMATION:

Overweight and Facing Blood Pressure Medication to Buffed and Perfect BP

Dieting was nothing new to me: During my twenty-seven years of marriage and raising two daughters, both now in their mid-twenties, the word *diet* was nothing new to me. Looking back, it seems as though someone in my family was always trying to lose weight with the latest popular "thin is in" craze. I lived through Richard Simmons's "Sweatin' to the Oldies," something called Scarsdale, whatever Oprah did, and who can forget adding up untold numbers of points printed on wrappers and labels. There was even the "Cabbage Soup" diet that landed my wife in the emergency room after losing twenty pounds in three weeks. Of course, none of these worked long term, and the lasting effects of failure just seem to add to a person's low self-esteem. It was a vicious cycle.

I didn't want to take blood pressure medication: A few months back, I sat at my desk wondering what I was going to do. I was fifty pounds overweight and looking at starting blood pressure medication. I didn't want to go on a prescription drug, so it looked like it was my turn to give this "diet" thing a whirl.

JIM BEFORE

JIM AFTER

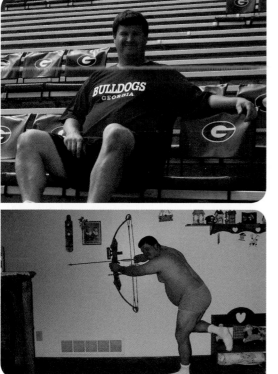

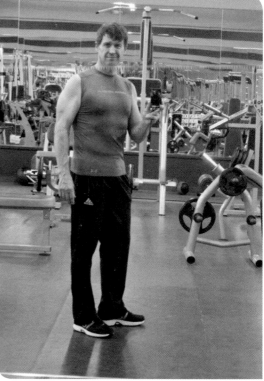

Timing is everything: For some reason that only Facebook knows, a blog with a fitness model in it appeared on my page. I must admit, the great-looking model is what first captured my attention, but after reading her blog explaining the proper nutrition and the hard work getting in shape was going to involve, Natalie Jill struck a chord with me. A no-excuse, work hard, and sweat-it-off program was something I could do. The word *diet* just sent shivers up my back, but Natalie seemed to concentrate more on what a person *can* eat, not what they *can't* eat. She was offering so much information and seemed genuinely concerned. I bought her *Stay Lean Recipes*, and it was *game on.*

Falling in love with unprocessing my diet: I subscribed to Natalie Jill's Facebook site and devoured everything I could about what she was doing. I watched her videos on YouTube. I fell in love with the "eat clean and natural" program. I learned the benefits of lifting weights and resistance training and started working out three times a week, allowing for a day of recovery between each visit to the gym. Days I did not go to the gym I did some yoga. Time in front of the TV was eliminated almost completely and replaced with reading and researching what I was doing. I was over the top, and my family had no choice but to come on board.

The family joined in: It's true—results are what matter, and that's what people see. I am eating natural, real unprocessed foods and enjoying it! My wife and my youngest daughter joined me after I had lost 20 pounds in the first two months. They were tired of counting points on candy bars and other processed foods. I am now 17 weeks in and down 43 pounds. My wife and daughter have both lost between 15 and 20 pounds. It is amazing to see what it has done for the self-image of each one of us! My blood pressure has dropped 25 to 30 points and is now well below the 120/80 standard. It's a lifestyle now, a habit.

Learning about my food: I learned about the different kinds of protein, carbohydrates, and fats and how to make them work together. Understanding these nutritional guidelines gave me confidence that I was doing the right thing. Food prep is something we now do together as a family. We prep 80 percent of our food for the week on the weekends, so instead of packaged processed foods, our refrigerator is filled with real food ready to eat. I learned to read labels and look up the ingredients. Learning what's in a lot of today's food is a real eye-opener! The support of Natalie Jill and her friends on Facebook has really helped. I love to read the posts and know there are others out there going through what I'm going through!

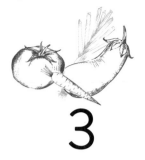

3

UNPROCESSING YOUR DIET— GOING BEYOND GLUTEN-FREE

"Little things done over time make a big *difference."*

I *do not* endorse a gluten-free diet as a method of losing weight. What I do endorse as a solid weight-loss method, is a nutrition plan free of processed food. Gluten-free eating has become a big trend, and we're seeing gluten-free this, that, and everything else in grocery stores, restaurants, and on school menus. But many of these items are still processed.

If you're wondering, "Should I go gluten-free?" the question you might ask yourself (assuming you're not a celiac or gluten intolerant) is, "Should I be eating an unprocessed diet?" Why? *Because eating an unprocessed diet is the healthiest way of eating on the planet,* the way people naturally ate for thousands and thousands of years. *Remember, every naturally unprocessed food on the planet is gluten-free* (wheat, barley, and rye—all containing gluten—are grains that have to be processed before they are consumed). As we'll see, a gluten-free diet isn't necessarily a healthy diet, especially if it is made up of gluten-free processed foods such as doughnuts, cupcakes, pasta, and more. For me, giving up gluten was the first step toward losing weight and enjoying better health. Unprocessing your diet is the way to go!

WHAT EXACTLY IS GLUTEN—AND WHAT DOES IT HAVE TO DO WITH PROCESSED FOODS?

First off, let's talk about what gluten is and why it is harmful. Then we'll take gluten-free to the next step: unprocessing your diet, so you can reach your ultimate health and weight goals.

Gluten is the protein found in wheat (all forms, including bulgur, durum, semolina, spelt, and so on), barley, and rye, as well as triticale (a wheat-rye hybrid—it's not very common, but it's important to be aware of if you happen to bump into it). Gluten gives dough its elasticity and helps foods such as bread keep their shape. It acts like a "glue" that holds them together, but it can also be found in unsuspecting foods from candy to soup to deli meats, as mass food manufacturers use it to thicken, stabilize, and emulsify many products. This is why you'll find it in so many processed foods.

Why would a person go gluten-free? There are two main reasons, and a third less obvious reason—one that goes beyond true intolerance and food trends. This third reason is the one that has been changing the lives of thousands of my followers.

1. You have celiac disease. With this autoimmune disorder, the body doesn't recognize gluten and can't digest it properly. The body responds in many ways, including with severe stomach pains and skin rashes serious enough for trips to the hospital, with progressively worsening symptoms. The only way to alleviate the symptoms of celiac disease is to completely remove gluten from the diet.

2. You are gluten intolerant. This just means your body doesn't do well with gluten (in the way that someone who is lactose intolerant doesn't do well with dairy), with symptoms such as bloating, stomachache, and fatigue that occur when you eat gluten. By eliminating gluten, these symptoms will likely be alleviated, but if you are gluten-free and eating a processed food diet, you may be left wondering why you're still having health and weight issues. I do not endorse a gluten-free diet on its own for losing weight.

3. You want to unprocess your diet (and feel and look like a million bucks!). Any naturally unprocessed food is gluten-free (see the definition below). So when you're eating an unprocessed diet, you're by default eating gluten-free, and an unprocessed food diet is better for everyone *no matter who you are.* And with the fabulous unprocessed gluten-free recipes included in this book, you'll find that going unprocessed and gluten-free is easy and delicious!

LET'S START UNPROCESSING!

This is so much easier than it sounds—you just have to put a little effort into it! Unprocessing your diet isn't about how the food is prepared or whether you have to cook it; it's about reducing or eliminating anything that's been chemically altered, often using artificial ingredients that the body doesn't even recognize as actual nutrients.

GLUTEN-FREE AND GAINING WEIGHT

ARE you on a gluten-free diet "just to lose weight" but are actually *gaining* weight? Many of us assume eliminating gluten is a free pass to weight loss, but if you're eating a processed gluten-free diet, this is far from the truth.

Did you know that many gluten-free baked foods are actually more fattening than those that contain gluten? The reason: wheat flour is often replaced with lower fiber, higher glycemic flours such as corn, tapioca, potato, or rice flours, which means the sugar and often the calorie content actually goes up! What's more, these high-sugar starches are absorbed into your bloodstream very quickly. This, in turn, causes your body to react with an insulin spike, which makes you crave more sugar and become hungrier—not to mention the artificial additives often found in gluten-free foods that are wreaking havoc with your health.

Since I was first diagnosed with celiac disease over a decade ago, a host of processed foods have popped up under the gluten-free label, so a cookie or a cracker that is gluten-free will likely still have a lot of junk inside, and is often highly processed.

The takeaway: never assume that gluten-free products are healthier for you. Skip the substitute flours and stick with whole foods on my unprocessed, gluten-free 7 Day Jump Start and you'll naturally start shedding the pounds. For many of us, giving up gluten is a necessity. But for many more still, it's not until we truly unprocess our diets that we begin to really lose weight and enjoy improved health.

For the sake of definitions, "processed food" is food that has been modified (by procedures such as extraction) or contains ingredients not occurring naturally. Processed foods range from grains that are moderately processed in order that they may be consumed to foods containing ingredients not found in nature. If you can't pronounce it or don't know what it is, odds are it is not a natural food. "Fat-free" and "artificially sweetened" products are not natural, and they can sabotage your health and weight-loss efforts. Heavily processed foods typically have little to no nutritional value and are loaded with empty calories. They do a great job of appealing to both our wallets and our taste buds, while hiding some potentially nasty ingredients that can do our bodies more harm than good. Simply put, heavily processed foods are a cheap and easy way to pollute your body.

On the flipside, an unprocessed diet is based on eating foods in their natural state without a whole lot of ingredients on the label (often just one ingredient!). An unprocessed diet is by nature gluten-free, assuming nothing has been added to it.

A rule of thumb: an unprocessed food is one that came from a plant, an animal, the ground, or the ocean. Think about what was available to our ancestors: nuts, seeds, plants, fruits, meat, poultry, and fish. These unprocessed foods should make up the bulk of your diet, but you could add some minimally processed grains and dairy if you like.

These three principles are all you need to remember to gauge whether a food is processed or unprocessed:

3 PRINCIPLES OF UNPROCESSED EATING

1. Eat foods that once grew. Any food that once grew—fruits, vegetables, nuts, seeds, meat, seafood—is unprocessed and is better for you than anything that didn't. Our prehistoric ancestors depended on these foods in the right proportions. If these nourishing foods were good enough for them, they're fine for you, too. Whole grains including brown rice, quinoa, oats and unprocessed dairy are fine in smaller amounts.

2. Remember the 10,000 years rule. If it was on this planet 10,000 years ago—think meats, fish and seafood, vegetables, fruits, nuts, and oils—it's probably great to eat. Corn syrup, artificial sweeteners, trans fats, and packaged foods were *not* here!

3. Eat real foods. If you can't pronounce the ingredients, put it back! If it has three ingredients, it's likely to be better for you than if it has fifty. A third grader should be able to read a label and know what is in the product.

UNPROCESSING IS ABOUT ADDING, NOT SUBTRACTING

The benefits to unprocessing your diet are indisputable. Every person in the world would do better with an unprocessed diet. Eating real, unprocessed food gives you abundant energy, keeps your blood sugar in check (because you're not eating a lot of processed starches and sugars), and helps you feel better all around. Plus, when you are eating real food, it is *a lot* harder to make poor choices and overeat. Making an unprocessed diet your lifestyle is the most effective way of losing weight and keeping it off for the long term. A healthy lifestyle is the only thing that lasts!

Unprocessing your diet means you'll be getting a good balance of nutrients based on clean food. I like to think of it as adding rather than subtracting: adding in a balance of healthy proteins, carbs, and fats through natural foods. If you're leaving less room for the junk, you're going to crave less of the junk. And you'll learn to appreciate the natural flavors of real food. So you end up with more energy, you lose a lot of that bloat, and you start feeling better. You will get to the point where it isn't "work" anymore. As I have found over and over, once people start feeling better, they want to keep going! And there's nothing better than feeling good to jump start your new healthy lifestyle and weight loss!

UNPROCESSING SUGAR FROM YOUR DIET

An unprocessed foods diet avoids added sugar, though it isn't a strict no-sugar or no-carb diet. Your body, and especially your brain, needs carbs to function. We just want to get our carbs the way nature intended, not from eating and drinking foods laden with added table sugar and artificial sweeteners.

But wait a minute—are we talking about carbs or sugar here? Actually, both. In reality, whether it's celery, spinach, fruit, or cupcakes, all carbs are ultimately sugars. Clearly you want to gravitate to the celery-type sugars over the cupcake sugars! But what I really want you to be aware of is the *added* sugar—table sugar—that so many people go crazy with. It's hidden in places you may not even be aware of. Take applesauce, for example. People think they're eating a healthy food when they open a jar of applesauce, but they might not realize just how much sugar it contains unless the brand they pick has "no sugar added." When you throw in an extra 20 grams of sugar to "regular" applesauce, that's where you're going to run into trouble. Unsweetened applesauce, the only kind I get, is naturally sweet from the apples and contains all the sugar you really want to put into your body (and if you're looking for an easy homemade recipe for applesauce, check out page 103).

Another place to look out for hidden sugar is fruit juice. This is one area that catches a lot of people. They feel like drinking fruit juice is a healthy thing to do, but in reality they may be doing themselves a big disservice. Now, fruit is healthy and we all should be eating some fruit every day. The problem is when that fruit is processed into juice. Think of it this way: the typical 8-ounce glass of apple juice has about 4 apples in it; you can drink 4 apples worth of sugar in less time than it would take to *eat* half of an apple! The body has a much different response to eating a single piece of fruit with all of its skin, pulp, and fiber intact than it does when you drink the equivalent of 4 to 10 pieces of fruit. Some very popular juice drinks will even tell you how much fruit is in the bottle. If you had to *eat* all of that fruit, it would be a next-to-impossible chore.

People are always asking me if I ever eat dessert. Sure, I've made room for the occasional "treat" (and yes, I do eat chocolate!) because we're all human and we all need a little indulgence in our lives. In my experience, any overly strict diet is more likely to fail, as it relies on willpower and deprivation—two things that are impossible to maintain in the long term. When I do enjoy a treat, I eat something that's real. For example, the recipes in the dessert section, from chia seed pudding to strawberry chocolate cobbler, feature my favorite real sweeteners, including fruit, honey, maple syrup, agave nectar, coconut nectar, and stevia. And I will have a scoop of *real* ice cream from time to time. Not the low-carb or any other highly processed kind, but pure ice cream with four ingredients—cream, milk, egg yolks, and sugar. If you take a look at the labels of low-carb or reduced-fat ice cream, they read like a science experiment, not something you would want to eat.

WHAT ABOUT SUGAR SUBSTITUTES?

Artificial sweeteners are a dieter's secret enemy. Many of my followers report that they rely on sugar substitutes to stay sugar-free but still crave sweets. Why? The theory is that our bodies sense the sweetness of the food and expect the calories. When you don't get those calories, your body still craves them, so you end up eating more calories elsewhere to make up for it, pushing you further away from your health and fitness goals. For example, if you eat fifteen sugar-free cookies, you'd be eating more sugar (and you still might want more, especially if those cookies are low fat!) than if you had eaten just two sugar-sweetened cookies.

The other big issue is that most artificial sweeteners are 200 to 600 times sweeter than sugar, and this can really mess with your taste buds! When you consume foods and beverages loaded with artificial sweeteners, you are training your taste buds to expect this sweetness. Then when you go to eat a naturally sweet food like berries, they no longer taste sweet because your palate is accustomed to foods that are 200 to 600 times sweeter than berries!

Once you've quit the habit, you'll have a newfound appreciation for naturally sweet foods. My husband, Brooks, used to drink diet sodas years ago as a treat, but he challenged himself to cut out the artificial sweeteners for thirty days and see how he felt. The results were dramatic. His taste buds totally changed, real food tasted better to him, and those artificial sweeteners became completely unappealing. The effect of artificial sweeteners on your body is truly amazing. They might not have calories, but they do make you want to keep eating artificially flavored foods. By going the thirty days without diet sodas, and unprocessing his diet, Brooks no longer needs extra willpower to stay away from those diet sodas.

One sugar substitute I get asked about a lot is stevia. This natural South American herb plant has been used for centuries to sweeten tea and other foods, and is considered the sugar substitute of the organic and natural foods industry. You can find it in liquid or powder form or fresh from the plant. Stevia has negligible effects on blood sugar and is useful to diabetics and those on unprocessed diets (that's you!).

Xylitol is another naturally occurring sweetener you might see as well. It looks and tastes like sugar but contains about 40 percent fewer calories than sugar and doesn't have a negative effect on blood sugar. Xylitol-sweetened foods are fine to eat in small amounts, but don't overdo it, as excess can cause gastrointestinal issues in some people.

Keep this in mind: real sugar contains just 15 calories a teaspoon and 45 calories a tablespoon. So when you'd like something a little sweet, I'd rather have you reach for a little real sugar or another natural sweetener than the artificial stuff.

IS DAIRY PART OF AN UNPROCESSED DIET?

When I was growing up, you'd see celebrity athletes, actors, and supermodels in commercials and ads wearing milk mustaches and

WITHDRAWAL FROM SUGAR AND OTHER PROCESSED FOODS

REMEMBER our first transformation, Joan (page 16), who drank four to five Mountain Dews for more than two decades? If she could quit the habit, you can, too! Some of us, like Joan, go through "withdrawal," whether it's from diet soda, sugar, or processed carbs, and the symptoms tend to be more intense the more there is to give up. You may feel tired or downright exhausted for a bit; you may be irritable and feeling a little down without all that artificial food stimulation (but you also skip the inevitable crash). Know that no matter how difficult it is at first, it will pass, and for most of us, pretty quickly. If you're craving sugar, turn to page 94 for tips on how to keep from giving in. And eating a balance of healthy protein, fats, and carbohydrates as part of the 7 Day Jump Start will give your body a new foundation to come through to the other side feeling better than ever. You can do this!

HIGH-FRUCTOSE CORN SYRUP—IT DOESN'T GET MORE ARTIFICIAL THAN THIS!

WHAT if you could manufacture a product that doesn't exist in nature anywhere, that's cheaper than sugar, sweeter than sugar, and causes an addictive reaction in whatever food it's used in so that you want to keep eating it? It's a mass food manufacturer's dream come true, and chances are you've been eating it for years!

High-fructose corn syrup (HFCS) is used as an additive in most processed foods and beverages including breads, cereals, breakfast bars, lunch meats, yogurt, soups, and condiments. The manufacturing process begins with corn, but the corn kernels are broken down and combined with three enzymes (alpha-amylase, glucoamylase, xylose isomerase) and spun at high speeds until a thick syrup forms. This enzymatic processing converts some of its glucose to fructose, making it a sweeter concoction of about 24 percent water and 76 percent sugars.

HFCS is used by manufacturers to create food that is cheap and easy to produce, easy to transport, and it lasts for an unrealistic amount of time on grocery store shelves. But think about your favorite foods, and especially baked goods—they are supposed to have a limited life in the cabinet or refrigerator, and they might turn out a little different each time you make them.

What's even scarier than the extended shelf life is what HFCS does to your body when you eat it. HFCS directly interferes with the metabolic process of leptin secretion in the body. Leptin is a critical hormone directly involved in the signals your body sends to indicate fullness. HFCS slows leptin secretion significantly, which leads to overeating and is a real challenge for anyone trying to moderate caloric intake.

From there it's a downward spiral. Cheap food that tastes good leads to overconsumption, which leads to increased chances for weight gain, metabolic syndrome, type 2 diabetes, and heart disease. So do what I do and stay away from HFCS. Read your food labels so you can be a smarter and healthier consumer!

asking "Got Milk?" Parents, teachers, *everyone* was saying, "If you want to be healthy, have strong bones and big muscles, you have to drink your milk!" Dairy products are commonly accepted as loaded with essential nutrients including protein, calcium, potassium, magnesium, folate, B vitamins, and vitamins A, D, and E. But lately, there has been a lot of buzz about eliminating dairy from our diets completely.

What happened? Well, the simple truth is that humans really aren't designed to consume dairy—we actually are the only mammals who do consume the milk of other mammals after childhood. And certain populations are generally intolerant of dairy. Take that, and add to it the fact that dairy processing has changed tremendously over the past few decades. Conventional (nonorganic) dairy farms have become big business. Cows and livestock are fed grains that are often genetically modified—not exactly the natural diet of cows. In nature, cows eat grass, not corn and other refined grains. Not only that, many cows are given antibiotics to keep them from getting sick from the filth and feces they stand in all day as they are packed into confined spaces, where they are eating the grains used to plump them up. To make things worse, they are fed growth hormones to make them bigger faster.

High calorie and fat content used to be the biggest complaints about dairy products, but as you can see, if you feed cows food that is not natural to them and load them up with hormones and antibiotics, the milk they produce will have the same by-products in it. That is why I always try to get my dairy from grass-fed, hormone-free cows.

LOWER LACTOSE AND DAIRY-FREE OPTIONS

Many people now suffer from lactose intolerance, meaning their bodies don't produce the enzymes to break down the sugars in dairy products, so the foods move into the colon, where they turn into bacteria. (In contrast, an allergy to dairy is usually severe and diagnosed in early childhood.) And as it turns out, many people who have celiac disease also are lactose intolerant. Symptoms of lactose intolerance include gas, abdominal cramping, and diarrhea. Luckily, there are now a variety of lactose-free dairy foods, and goat's milk cheeses are lower in lactose than those made from cow's milk and thus more digestible for some. You may do well with yogurt, which is a fermented dairy product. Look for the "live and active cultures" seal; these active cultures help break down the lactose in the food so some people with lactose intolerance can eat them. The good news is that some people may be able to tolerate dairy again once they manage to repair their gut.

Worldwide studies are being conducted to prove the health benefits of live and active cultures found in yogurt (those super-food probiotics that everyone's talking about), including preventing gastrointestinal infections, boosting the body's immune system, fighting certain types of cancer, and preventing osteoporosis. Greek-style yogurt is one of my favorites because it's high in protein and low in calories and sugar. Make sure your yogurt is unsweetened, as commercial flavored yogurts pack in the sugar as well as a host of artificial sweeteners and fillers. Yogurt should have, more or less two ingredients: milk and live active cultures. These live active cultures—the probiotics that are found naturally in the fermented dairy—are so important for your digestion and overall health.

Kefir, a fermented milk beverage—yogurt's drinkable cousin—is another probiotic-rich form of dairy. Its flavor is refreshingly tangy, and it has a slight effervescence to it. Like yogurt, its live and active cultures make it more digestible for some who are sensitive to dairy. And as with yogurt, look for the words "contains live active cultures" on the label, and stay away from flavored (i.e., sweetened) kefir.

If you go dairy-free, be conscious of hidden dairy. Dairy by-products including curds, whey, casein, rennet, and lactose are found in many foods and beverages, so read your labels carefully and look for the words "dairy-free" on the label to be sure.

For dairy-free milk, I favor unsweetened almond milk and coconut milk; they are typically fortified with calcium, so your body won't miss the calcium from the dairy. Just make sure to read labels—with so many brands to choose from, yours should be one with no added sugar or additives. I avoid nondairy milks containing the thickener carrageenan—this seaweed derivative can tend to cause bloating and digestive issues in some people. Other calcium-rich foods include figs, Brazil nuts, hazelnuts, broccoli, cabbage, kelp, dark leafy greens (such as bok choy, kale, mustard greens, collard greens, and turnip greens), and seafood (such as oysters and salmon).

If you choose to include dairy in your diet, that's fine. Just remember to make the healthiest dairy choices possible. Stay mindful of portion sizes, calories, and especially added sugar content. At a minimum, make sure you are buying full-fat dairy that is BST (growth hormone)-free dairy.

EAT LIKE A CAVEMAN (OR CAVEWOMAN)

My plan has a lot in common with the popular Paleo diets, but with a strong emphasis on plant-based foods. While abundant vegetables are a core part of my plan, healthy meats are also included, which is why I tell my followers to "Eat like a caveman or cavewoman."

I also recognize that a healthy unprocessed foods diet can contain some grains—just make sure those grains are unrefined and gluten-free. Quinoa, whole-grain rice, and gluten-free oats, as well as some dairy can be enjoyed in moderation, which makes my lifestyle nutrition program easier to follow than a strict Paleo diet.

On the plan, I recommend eating two servings of starchy carbs a day, with the rest of your carbs coming from fruits and vegetables. Once you get to the point where you're

KISS (KEEP IT SUPER SIMPLE)

DO these three things, and over time you will be in shape:

1. Just move! Walk, walk, and walk some more. It doesn't have to be scheduled; just make a point to walk more during the day. Park farther away, take "long-cuts," use the stairs, take walking breaks at work, walk after lunch—whatever you can fit in. See page 240 to learn why sitting is the new smoking. It's no joke!

2. Drink water! It doesn't get much simpler than that. Nor does it get more important, which is why I'll continue to remind you to stay hydrated. Our bodies are 70 percent water, and you need more water to burn body fat. Add sliced organic lemon or cucumber for flavor if you like. Swapping just one 12-ounce soda or fruit juice for water each day will save you about 10 to 15 pounds over the course of a year!

3. Small plates! Portion control is key. Eat your meals on salad plates and use small bowls for cereal, soups, and desserts. Trick your mind. A "full" small plate looks better than the same food on a large plate with empty space.

close to your goal weight, you'll be able to add more carbs back in. Then, once you're maintaining that goal weight, you'll never have to diet again! You'll be able to have the occasional treat—just not every day. When you do enjoy those treats, your body won't mind because the rest of the time you'll be nourishing it with the healthiest food on earth. The more committed you are to un-processing—treat days included—the better you'll feel, and that's my sole purpose with this program!

MAJORITY RULES

Once you make this your lifestyle, if you do what's right *most* of the time, you won't have to worry too much about having a sweet treat or a treat meal on occasion.

But before we get too far, I want to make sure we're clear on a few things. This is about a lifestyle, and maintaining is a lot easier than losing. If you want to lose weight, I want you to follow the 7 Day Jump Start exactly as written for at least one week, and possibly longer depending on how much you have to lose. One thing I see all the time is that when people start to lose weight, they start to "coast," thinking they will keep losing. They usually get a reality check that reminds them they have to stick with it. In the end, by making it your lifestyle, you will never look back.

It takes seventeen to thirty days to change an old habit and create a new one, so I really want you to keep going after you jump start things the first week. I want you to be strict with yourself at first, as you need to turn those habits into your lifestyle. You truly need to feel the true benefits of eating this way. Then you can start having a treat meal here and there. But remember, this is a treat, not a green light to stuff yourself silly. Don't go crazy with the portions—eat mindfully and enjoy every bite—and eat the real thing. Have a doughnut, not the box of twelve. Have a bowl of ice cream, not the entire carton. Have a slice or two of pizza, not the entire pie. If you go off with fake alternatives, you won't be satisfied—you'll still crave the real deal.

Now when I tell you that the most important part of this program involves cutting out processed foods, you know just what that means. This single lifestyle change is the one that will give you long-term results so you'll never have to "diet" again!

10 FOUNDATIONS OF A FIT LIFESTYLE

1. Stay hydrated and drink water throughout the day.
2. Look for opportunities to walk during the day.
3. Eat vegetables every day.
4. Eat a balance of protein, fat, and carbohydrates at every meal.
5. Watch your portion sizes.
6. Eat real, unprocessed foods that you can define.
7. Eliminate hydrogenated oils, corn syrup, artificial sweeteners, and other ingredients you can't pronounce.
8. Challenge yourself physically every day.
9. Look for solutions, not excuses.
10. Take responsibility for your health and well-being.

RACHEL BEFORE

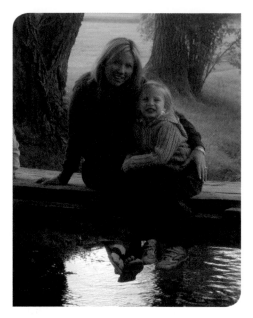

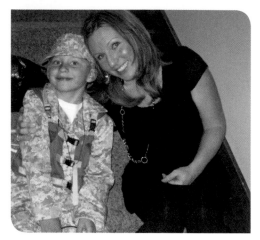

RACHEL AFTER

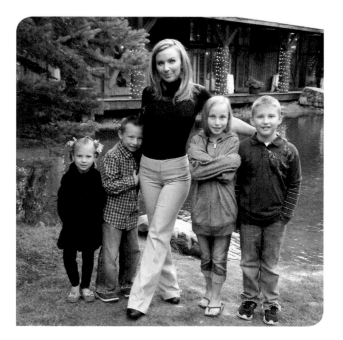

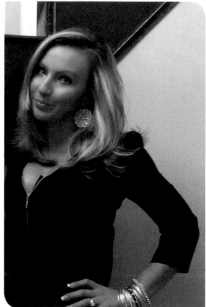

RACHEL'S TRANSFORMATION:

From Cookie-Baking Mother of Four to Launching Clean Food Crush

Baking cookies like any "good mom": When I found Natalie's program, I had given birth to four kids within five years. My entire life was focused on the kids. I loved cooking and baking, so I'd watch cooking shows and make the treats I'd see moms putting together on TV. I thought I was being a good mom by baking cookies almost every day and cooking hugely fattening casseroles. But my family was eating too much sugar and too much processed food. I didn't know the difference, because that's how I grew up and that's just what we did.

Feeling horrible: The problem with all those cookies was that I was feeling horrible. At first I thought that's just what happens when you get older—after all, I had just had four kids. I felt that I was doing things the right way, but I had gained so much weight and didn't recognize my body anymore. My body had been through a lot!

Time for a change: When I came across Natalie's program online, it sounded amazing and looked like exactly what I needed. I knew it was time for a change. I wondered if I could really follow through with the plan. I immediately ordered her program and downloaded it, and the next day I did the food shopping. I followed the program to a T.

Losing 30 pounds by Christmas: In the first week of the program, I already could put on smaller pants because of all the water weight I had lost. That gave me the motivation to keep going. It was September, and literally by the holidays, my body had completely changed. I was working out, and I had lost all 30 pounds by Christmastime. I couldn't believe it was possible. I looked better than even I had before I had my children. Friends started noticing immediately. They would ask, "What in the world are you doing?" "Are you eating?" I answered that I was, in fact, eating plenty of food, and often. It was all about *what* I was eating. I realized that there was a better way of doing things.

Launching a clean food blog: Over the next year I started experimenting more and more with this new way of eating, making familiar recipes healthier and creating my own recipes. I found that using natural ingredients was easier than I thought. I changed the way I cooked for my family and me, and my kids loved it! I started sharing recipes online here and there, and it really took off. Over the next few years, my second transformation occurred, with the launch of my blog, Clean Food Crush, an amazing dream business. None of this would have ever happened without Natalie. Natalie is one of those completely generous people who just wants to help others to succeed. I thought, "She's a mom, just like me. If she could do it, so could I." Finding the 7 Day Jump Start changed my life in so many ways and turned me into a happier, more energetic mom who is able to help other people. My whole family has benefited from eating better and by having a happier mother. I have so many dreams and goals, all sparked by Natalie's program!

4

PROTEIN, CARBS, AND FAT: THE 3 FOUNDATIONS OF THE 7 DAY JUMP START

"The goal: Never hungry, never full."

LET me introduce you to the 7 Day Jump Start's core building blocks—protein, carbohydrates, and fats, also known as macronutrients. While *macronutrient* isn't exactly the sexiest word you'll come across in this book, it's really important to get an understanding of these nutrients in order to learn how to build a balanced meal. Plus, our bodies depend on them for their very existence!

Macronutrients provide energy and are needed in large amounts because they are crucial to growth, metabolism, and basic functions (as opposed to micronutrients such as vitamins and minerals, which the body uses in smaller amounts).

My plan focuses on getting each of the macronutrients into your body in the proper amounts. Using the whole, fresh ingredients in the recipes I've included in this book, you'll be getting all the macronutrients you need every day in the perfect balance. I'll make it easy for you to put together a nourishing meal (see pages 83–93). And how will you know when you've had enough? Remember this motto: *"Never hungry, never full."*

Balance means you won't be restricting an entire category of macronutrient in an effort to lose weight. No more fat-free foods and diets, and no more focusing on low-carb or no-carb. These restriction-type diets provide short-term results at best and often are the start of yo-yo dieting as you restrict for a while and then let go, each time wreaking havoc on your body and metabolism. *Restricted diets are never a long-term solution.* Instead, we just need to focus on adding the right macronutrients to our body, focusing on *where* we're getting them and in *what form.*

"NEVER HUNGRY, NEVER FULL"

Stuffing yourself with anything is a bad idea—this means you're ignoring important signals and taking your body beyond what it actually needs. Likewise, you need enough food so your body can maintain and repair itself and promote the growth of lean muscle mass while minimizing fat storage. So if you're hungry, eat. But if you're full, put the fork down.

MEASURING SERVINGS WITHOUT A SCALE

A scale can come in handy in meal planning, but it's totally optional. To put together a meal with just the right amount of protein, fats, and carbs, all you really need is your hand!

Protein (cooked): the size of your palm or fist

Starchy carbs (cooked): the size of your palm or fist

Fats: the size of your thumb

And remember, vegetables are unlimited!

Now let's go over the benefits of these three critical macronutrients:

PROTEIN: FOR A LEAN, MEAN BODY

Protein plays a starring role in all of my nutrition plans. Coming in at 4 calories per gram, it is essential for growth and both building and maintaining lean muscle tissue, which, in turn, increases your metabolism. Protein contributes to the regulation of enzymes and hormones, to the structure of red blood cells, and the proper functioning of antibodies (which help you resist infection). If you're looking to get lean so you can have chiseled abs, say yes to protein!

Protein is the macronutrient that most women do not get enough of. Protein is very important for not only keeping your body satisfied and helping with lean mass, but is also key for healthy hair, skin, and nails! See, I knew *that* would help the ladies out there want to eat more protein! Not only that, but protein is especially important for women in order to maintain muscle mass and support bone density as we age.

The building blocks of proteins are amino acids, which are found in a variety of whole foods. Some foods contain more amino acids than others. Complete proteins have all of the essential amino acids and can be found in meat, poultry, fish, dairy, and eggs. Incomplete proteins (missing certain essential amino acids) can be found in foods such as nuts, nut butters, whole grains, legumes, beans, and certain vegetables. My general rule for protein portions is 4 to 6 ounces (depending on your sex and size), or the size of your palm or fist. See page 93 for a list of protein options available to you on the 7 Day Jump Start.

THE BENEFITS OF PROTEINS

- Directly involved in growth and tissue repair as well as preserving lean muscle tissue.
- Critical in making essential hormones and enzymes as well as in immune function.
- Helps the body secrete the hormone glucagon, which works to govern insulin and keep levels in check.
- Provides a secondary energy source when carbohydrates/glucose are no longer available.
- Supports growth of healthy skin, hair, and nails—if you like having nice skin, hair, and nails, make sure you get plenty of quality protein!

FATS: TO KEEP YOU FULL AND MAKE YOUR MEALS DELICIOUS

Fat really has gotten a bad rap, but hear this: fat is an important fuel source for the body, and, gram for gram, fat provides twice the energy of carbs or protein in the body. This is because dietary fat has 9 calories per gram—this is an important number because it's more than twice the calories (4) provided by 1 gram of carbohydrate or 1 gram of protein. See the Sidebar to see why those 9 calories are so important.

The key is the type of fat in just the right amount. How much fat is enough? I recommend including a small measure of fat in all your meals to fill you up and make your food more delicious. My general guideline is to use 1 tablespoon or an amount about the size of your thumb. A tablespoon might not seem very big, but if you take a tablespoon of olive oil and pour it over your salad, you'll see just how far it goes in making your veggies taste scrumptious. That may be reason alone to stop you from attacking that cheeseburger and fries!

Fat satisfies hunger and cravings, keeps you full longer, and can help raise HDL cholesterol, which is your good cholesterol. Eating healthy fats will actually help you manage your weight-loss efforts by providing a better sense of satiety than eating lower fat foods. It is much easier to avoid overeating when your body naturally tells you that you aren't hungry. That is why having healthy fats and protein in every meal is so key—it gives you a one-two punch to stop those cravings and help you feel full and satisfied. Fat is not the enemy, and it actually plays a pretty important role, especially if fat loss and being lean is your goal.

When you do not eat enough fat and you opt for a low-fat, high-carbohydrate diet, you will most likely feel hungrier and eat *more*, which will lead to weight gain. Remember the skinny on fat: eating fat will not make you fat!

Here's a thought: you'll be able to better manage your weight loss efforts when you actually *like* what you're eating! When you like what you're eating, it is easy to make it a lifestyle. See page 94 for a list of fat options available to you on the 7 Day Jump Start.

THE BENEFITS OF FATS

- Critical for growth and develop-ment, including maintaining cell membranes and providing cushion-ing for internal organs.
- Aid the body in absorbing certain vitamins, including vitamins A, D, E, K, and carotenoids.
- Lubricate joints.
- Maintain healthy skin and hair.
- Make food taste good.
- Help to curb cravings and provide a sense of fullness.

And don't forget the most delicious of fats, the avocado! Include it in your salads, add it as a side to any meal, and use it in your recipes. See pages 146, 153, 157, 198, 225 for just some of my favorite dishes using this wonderfully creamy fruit.

Note that I don't include peanuts as a nut option, for three reasons: 1) they are highly allergenic to many people; 2) they contain aflatoxin, a mold-produced toxin that's been found to be a carcinogen; and 3) they are not a true nut but rather a legume. That said, you can still get results on the program if you eat peanuts as your fat—the decision is yours to make.

FATS TO AVOID ON AN UNPROCESSED DIET:

Commercial (processed) mayonnaise
Vegetable shortening
Overly processed cheese (moderate amounts of real cheese are OK; goat's milk cheeses are my preferences, as they are lower in lactose)
Processed canola, corn, and soybean oil
Partially hydrogenated oils (the source of trans fats)

MY TOP 3 FATS

Coconut oil, olive oil, and butter (specifically, clarified butter or ghee) are the fats you'll find in almost all my recipes, and the ones I favor in every meal I prepare. Let's learn a lit-tle about the three.

Coconut Oil

If you haven't used coconut oil before, you are in for a treat! Coconut oil not only tastes great, but it is a high-temperature oil, mean-ing it can be heated to higher temperatures than other vegetable oils without breaking down, making it ideal for cooking. I love to use it in my stir-fries. It's also great added to baked goods such as cookies and brownies for a nutritional boost and added flavor.

NOT ALL FATS ARE CREATED EQUAL

CURRENT research shows that both saturated fats, like butter and coconut oil, and unsaturated fats, like olive oil, play a role in a healthy diet. These three fats happen to be my favorites (see more on them below)! I also recommend including generous amounts of heart-healthy omega-3 fatty acid–rich fish in your diet (vegetarians can get their omega-3s from flax and chia seeds).

But while all fats contain the same amount of calories, not all fats are created equal. Canola, corn, and soybean oil (aka vegetable oil) are fats that I do not recommend, as they are often processed and heavily refined. An oil should taste like the food it came from; if a fat has no taste, as in the case of canola oil, chances are its flavor and aroma have been stripped out in a chemical and high-heat process that denatures the heat-sensitive fatty acids. These oils become processed, contribute to the formation of free radicals, and thus are potentially carcinogenic and have no place in an unprocessed diet.

The worst type of fats—the ones that I try to always avoid—are trans fats. Trans fats are found naturally in some foods including meat, butter, and milk, which are not a problem, but most come from foods containing partially hydrogenated oil. For the most part, trans fats are solid rather than liquid at room temperature. The process of partial hydrogenation makes the oils easier to cook with and less likely to spoil. It's also a cheap way of manufacturing fats that processed food manufacturers love. Trans fats give your cardiovascular system a double whammy, both raising your LDL ("bad") cholesterol and lowering your HDL ("good") cholesterol. Trans fats are directly linked to heart disease.

Since 2006, the U.S. Food and Drug Administration has required food manufacturers to list trans fat content as a separate line on nutrition labels. This has led to a reduction in the use of trans fats, and in some places governments have banned the use of trans fats in restaurant foods. While these fake fats are making their way out of the food supply, beware of the cheap refined vegetable oils that have been taking their place—they have *no* place in an unprocessed diet!

FATS IN YOUR HEALTHY DIET INCLUDE:

Nuts (unsalted and raw)	Nut butters	Seeds	Cooking fats
almonds	almond	chia	butter/clarified butter (see page 49 for more info.)
cashews	cashew	flax	coconut oil (unrefined)
Brazil nuts	walnut	hemp	olive oil
macadamia nuts		pumpkin	sesame
pecans			
walnuts			

REMEMBER THE WAR AGAINST FAT?

FLASH back to the Eighties: Scrunchies, leg warmers, Jane Fonda workouts, and Richard Simmons aerobics classes were all the rage, along with fat-free gummy bears, "low-fat" snack foods, and more. Fat was the enemy. We thought everything was healthy as long as it was labeled "fat-free" or "low-fat." We all firmly believed the new government mantra that dietary fat was the enemy.

Meanwhile, junk food manufacturers were subbing in extra sugar and simple carbs for the fat, and, suddenly, we found ourselves smack in the middle of an obesity epidemic. Why? Without fat, we tend to feel hungrier, more sluggish, and we have less energy. As a result, we'll tend to exercise less and are more likely to binge. This is made even worse when bingeing on fat-free (read: processed) treats that don't fill you up and just lead to eating even more.

Although we became fatter as a nation by banishing fat, the fear of fat has lingered on in some circles, even as science has proven that fat is *not* the enemy it was once thought to be. I have received quite a few emails over the past few years from people who thought they would "speed up" their results by cutting out the fat, only to find out the exact opposite the hard way. So please don't be afraid of fats. They are a very necessary part of losing weight and staying lean.

Consider this: Eating fat will not make you fat. What does make you fat is:

1. Eating more calories than your body uses
2. Eating empty calories with no nutritional value
3. Eating too many refined carbohydrates and sugars
4. Not getting the appropriate balance of fats, carbs, and proteins
5. Living a sedentary lifestyle (i.e. being a couch potato)
6. Not working out

Coconut oil can be part of a healthy weight-loss plan. Most of its fat comes from medium-chain triglycerides in the form of lauric acid, which the body uses as energy. Think of it as a fat that the body uses for energy like a carb. Lauric acid also increases good (HDL) cholesterol in our blood, which improves ratios of HDL and LDL cholesterol, making it a heart-healthy oil. There is also evidence that coconut oil reduces inflammation, boosts energy and endurance, and improves digestion and absorption of other nutrients including vitamins and amino acids. In addition, coconut oil positively affects blood sugar and can boost thyroid function, leading to increased metabolism. Coconut oil contains antifungal, antibacterial, and antiviral properties. And there is even research supporting coconut oil's role in preventing wrinkles and age spots. In the world of super-foods, coconut oil is a super-fat!

Make sure to choose a coconut oil labeled as "unrefined" or "virgin" to avoid unknowingly purchasing a processed oil.

Olive Oil

Olives are one of the oldest foods known to humans. Olives are to olive oil like grapes are to wine, meaning the growing location and other variables that go into the production of olive oil yield dramatic differences in color, aroma, and flavor, just like grapes from different regions produce differences in wine. Extra virgin olive oil is the best quality (and least processed) and also the most expensive variety, as it comes from the first pressing of the olives. It is the least acidic and has the fruitiest flavor.

Extra virgin works great for salad dressings and is not meant to be a high-heat cooking oil. When heated above low to moderate temperatures, it loses many of its healthy benefits. I know a lot of people use olive oil to coat their pans when they're cooking, but you really should use coconut oil most of the time. Ideally, olive oil should be added to foods *after* they have been cooked. Olive oil is a monounsaturated oil with no cholesterol; it contains flavonoid polyphenols, which are natural antioxidants that have anti-inflammatory effects. Olive oil is a heart-healthy oil, best known for its role as the traditional fat of the Mediterranean diet, a staple for some of the world's healthiest people.

Butter

Yes, butter is a saturated fat, and yes, it's OK to eat! Current research has found no relationship between the intake of saturated fat and the incidence of heart disease and stroke. Remember, it's always better to eat a *real* food than a processed food, so watch out for trans fats and cheap vegetable oils, and enjoy butter as one of your fat choices.

Many of my recipes call for clarified butter, which is simply butter with the milk solids removed. When those milk solids are browned before removing them, it becomes ghee, a traditional fat used in Indian cooking that boasts a deliciously nutty taste. Ghee is rich in vitamins A, D, E, and K. (Side note: Ladies in India use ghee as a facial moisturizer and on their hair to make it strong and shiny.) Because the milk proteins are effectively removed from the butter to clarify it, many people who don't tolerate dairy are able to eat clarified butter and ghee.

To make clarified butter, melt butter slowly over low heat until the milk solids separate, then skim the foam off the top and pour the clarified butter into a container, leaving the milk solids behind. To go a step further and make ghee, continue to heat the butter until those milk solids turn brown before removing them. You can store jars of homemade ghee in the cupboard for up to three months (it doesn't require refrigeration). Jars of prepared ghee can be found in the grocery aisle of natural food stores and Indian groceries, so you don't have to make your own if you don't have the time.

One of the great things about clarified butter is that it has a higher smoke point (the point at which the oil begins to smoke, producing toxic fumes and harmful free radicals) than olive oil, making it great for higher-heat cooking. And you'll love its beautiful golden color—like liquid sunshine in a jar!

Carbohydrates: A Crucial Source of Fuel

Talk about a bad rap! Along with the low-fat craze, there was a low-carb craze. But going low- or no-carb is not a long-term solution to weight loss by any means. Learning about carbs—good and bad—and how to eat your carbs properly is very important to a healthy lifestyle. Carbohydrates are a major source of energy. At 4 calories per gram, carbs fuel our activities and are the main energy source for muscle function. The body breaks down carbohydrates to access glucose (a sugar) to be used for energy, and, in the process, also provide us with fiber, vitamins, and minerals.

Simple carbohydrates, often referred to as "bad carbs," are refined or processed foods that offer very little nutritional value. Examples of these are sugar, white bread, sugary cereals, and other highly processed foods that typically come in a box or a wrapper. They are digested quickly and easily by the body, causing rapid spikes in blood glucose levels, followed by rapid drops. The rise and fall of blood glucose triggers similar insulin spikes and drop-offs (ever had that tired sluggish feeling after a big pasta meal?) as a result. These insulin spikes have a negative impact on our weight-loss efforts. We want to keep insulin levels steady for the most part, avoiding big spikes and big crashes.

Complex carbohydrates, also known as "good carbs," are fiber-rich and digested much more slowly. Examples are whole grains, legumes, beans, seeds, many fruits, and starchy vegetables. This slow digestion process keeps blood glucose (and insulin levels) steady, offering our bodies more consistent energy to burn so that we can keep going.

Complex carbs keep us full longer and provide slow-burning energy, while simple carbs are the most easily consumed and turn to sugar in the body, which can wreak havoc on your weight-loss goals.

The best types of carbohydrates are the ones that are high in fiber and come primarily from vegetables and fruits. Gluten-free grains that are minimally processed are allowed on my plan, but you'll want to avoid refined grains completely until you are at your goal weight. At that time, if you want some pasta or other processed grain, it will be up to you to consume in moderation. For me, once I kick the habit with the "bad stuff," I don't like to open the door back up to it, as it can be a little too easy to slip back into old habits. I also include gluten-free bread as an option; just make sure you get the best quality possible with minimal ingredients.

Two of your carb servings can come from the starchy carb group and the third should be non-starchy. See page 62 for a list of starchy and non-starchy carbohydrates on the 7 Day Jump Start.

EATING A BALANCE OF PROTEIN, CARBS, AND FATS

A calorie is just a unit of measurement, and all calories are not created equal. You will not get the same results if you subsist on a diet of 1500 calories of gummy bears each day as you would by eating 1500 calories of healthy proteins, fats, and carbohydrates. Likewise, you will get completely different results from eating 1500 calories in one sitting as opposed to spreading out your calories throughout the day. You will not have the same energy, and you will not be working toward your long-term health goals.

There is much more to weight loss than just eating low-carb or low-fat, and that's why neither of those fads have worked well over time. Your body doesn't target just one type of calorie when it needs energy. When we burn calories during exercise, our bodies tap into stored glycogen (carbohydrates), fat, and sometimes protein (muscle). There's a definite process, and it all depends on what state your body is in. You can't consume 500 calories of junk and then assume you burned it all off because the treadmill said you did. Each one of the macronutrients behaves differently in the body, so it's critical that you understand your nutrition, not just count calories.

The key to weight loss, and how I designed my plan, is to create an environment in which you have the right balance of macronutrients (fats, carbs, protein) at all of your meals, so your body is nutritionally sound

THE BENEFITS OF CARBOHYDRATES

- The main source of fuel for the body, as they are easily accessible in the form of glucose. No fuel = no energy!
- Necessary for the brain, muscles, and central nervous system to function properly.
- Important for GI health and waste elimination.
- Include fiber, and a diet high in fiber has been directly linked to a decreased risk for obesity, heart disease, cholesterol, and certain types of cancer.

and can start burning off the excess body fat. By using the proper mix of foods, you will train your body to become efficient at using not only your food for energy, but also your stored body fat. You will be getting more nutrition for your body in fewer calories than you would by eating highly processed foods. You will be feeling satisfied and you will have plenty of energy to help you get through your daily activities and workouts effectively and safely.

GETTING INTO FAT-BURNING MODE

My program will put you in "fat-burning" mode, where you are firing up your metabolism and then stoking the fire throughout the day with healthy and delicious meals. It might be tempting to get "restrictive" and take your calorie count or fat or carb count even lower, thinking it will "speed up" the results. *Don't do that.* Not only will it not work, it will have the opposite effect. Your body is an amazing machine, and when it feels like you're starving it, it goes out of its way to conserve energy.

We want to get your metabolism revved up, not slow it down to a crawl. That is a dreaded catch-22 that I have seen with so many people. Their weight loss slows, so they keep eating less and less. This further slows their metabolism, so they eat even less, and by this point they think they are doomed. They are eating hardly any food yet not losing, and oftentimes even gaining, weight. Sound familiar? If so, you're probably wondering, "How is this possible?"

Simple: when you eat less and less, not only do you slow your metabolism, but your body starts burning muscle for fuel, and *not* body fat. Remember how body fat has 9 calories per gram? It has more than twice the energy of carbs and protein, which have 4 calories per gram. As a survival mechanism, the body wants to hold body fat as energy stores because it is going into "starvation mode." As the body turns to using your lean mass for energy, this further slows your metabolism. When you do eat your meal (at that point, most people are only eating one or two times per day because they are eating so few calories), the body can't process it all at one time because of the slowed-down metabolism. This excess is stored as body fat, while the body continues to burn muscle for energy. The only way out of this trap is to get your metabolism going again and start eating properly.

That is why this program isn't effective if your metabolic rate drops into economy mode, or worse, starvation mode, because it doesn't have enough fuel. So don't deviate from the nutrition plan I've provided. Make sure you include all three macronutrients in the course of your day and fulfill your nutritional needs with delicious whole foods! Fight the urge to cut out the fats or the carbs, thinking it will provide you with faster results. It will *not* work, and it will actually set you back. Focus on making it a lifestyle, and before you know it, you will be living a life full of energy and you won't have to worry about your next diet. You will be less stressed and much happier. I love it when people reach that lifestyle point!

LISI'S TRANSFORMATION:

From Shattered Bones to Healthy, Fit, and Bikini Ready

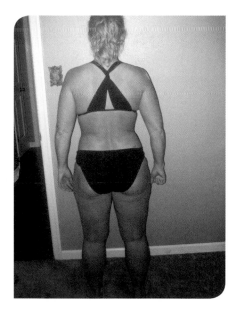

LISI BEFORE

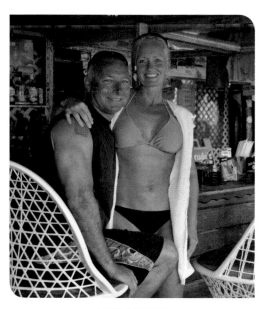

LISI AFTER

The trauma: In 2005 I was involved in a life-changing skiing accident that caused my left arm and oblique area to be completely paralyzed for three years. Before my accident, I worked in firefighting and arson investigation. It was a physically demanding job, and I was always in shape.

The weight gain: Over the course of my recovery, I gained 50 pounds. I was basically couch-ridden and couldn't leave the house except for my grueling physical therapy appointments. Diet and exercise were the furthest things from my mind, and eating convenience foods, drinking two liters or more of Diet Coke a day, and eating sugary desserts became the norm for me. Almost six years later, I had 80 percent usage of my left arm, but I will never be 100 percent because of the nerve damage. I began exercising again, but the weight was slow to come off. I was no longer able to run, swim, or lift weights like I had so easily done before, and this caused me to become depressed.

Hitting rock bottom: Soon after, I had a major setback—a tendon in my uninjured right wrist was damaged due to all of the strain I had been putting on my right arm. Two surgeries later, I regained some weight, could only get into sweatpants, and again fell back into the horrible eating habits of convenience foods and comfort foods. I was unable to work out for seven months.

Attempting fad diets: I knew things needed to change. I paid for two different meal-planning and exercise-planning industry "professionals," spending over a thousand dollars. I tried every fad diet from low-carb, prepackaged meals, and diets I read about in magazines to many different so-called weight-loss supplements, all with few results. I would wear pants and long-sleeve shirts all the time, even in the summer, because the way my body looked embarrassed me.

Finding the 7 Day Jump Start: Finally, I started to search the Internet for answers. That's when I discovered Natalie Jill's Facebook page. I read the testimonials and purchased her 7 Day Jump Start program. Something about it just seemed right to me. I weighed myself and I took measurements and photos. I was determined to make it work this time!

Seeing changes: The first week on the Jump Start, I felt great, and I lost 3 pounds! I kept at it, and more weight kept trickling off every week. After I lost 10 pounds, the scale didn't seem to be moving much, so I took photos again to compare them with my starting photos. I couldn't believe the difference; if my face had not been in those photos, I would have sworn they weren't photos of me.

Bikini time: I had a beach vacation planned for the spring, so that gave me a goal to work toward, and that was when I would take my after photos. When I took my photos four months after I had started, I couldn't believe the transformation my body had gone through! My body looked better than it had when I was in my twenties and working as a firefighter. And amazingly, the chronic nerve pain in my injured arm had diminished. I am certain that eliminating processed food was a big part of this improvement.

No magic pill: There is no secret pill or weight-loss scheme with Natalie. Her diet plan is truly a lifetime eating plan, not really a diet at all. I followed her plan by eating five to six meals a day. I ate only clean, gluten-free, sugar-free foods. I drank lots of water, took a multivitamin every day, and my Diet Coke addiction was history! My cravings eventually went away. I was never hungry, and some days it was hard to actually eat all of the food required. I would cook my meals for the week on Sunday, separate them into single servings, and when I got home from the gym, all I had to do was pull my dinner out of the fridge and heat it up. This left me no excuses for falling off track. If there is a secret to this plan, it is simply the clean eating and moderate exercise.

Energy—welcome back! Natalie's Jump Start plan gave me so much energy that I had to find things to keep me active. I started doing hot yoga every week, and I also did several high-intensity interval training (HIIT) sessions a week and some weight training. When Sunday came along, I would allow myself a cheat meal, which was usually pancakes, but as I got further along in the program I no longer even wanted a cheat meal. Now, unhealthy foods full of gluten and sugar make me feel awful. All I crave are clean healthy foods and water. Natalie has really been a godsend. If I can come back after major injuries and setbacks, then anyone can do it!

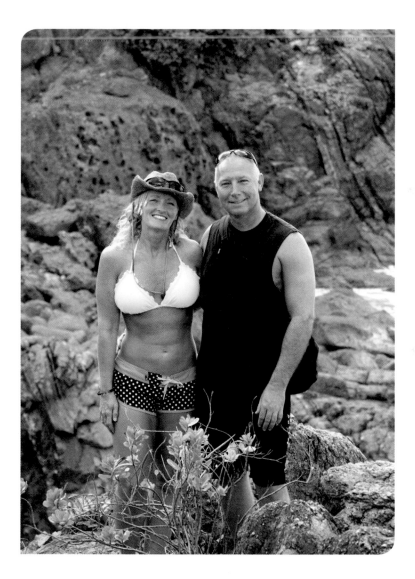

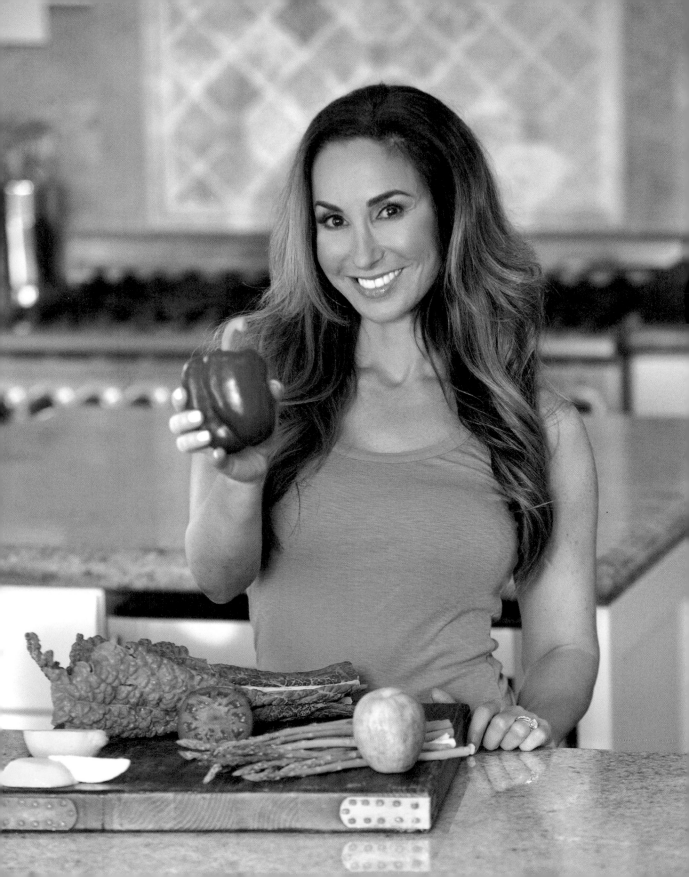

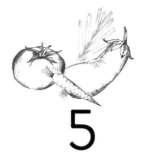

5

WHAT YOU'LL BE EATING
ON THE 7 DAY JUMP START—
THE GUIDELINES

"Decide. Commit. Live it, breathe it.
Do it. Not partway but all the way."

NOW that you've learned how simple and delicious unprocessing your diet can be, it's time to officially launch your 7 Day Jump Start! The program has really exciting recipes to keep your taste buds happy (pages 99 to 236) and exercise options that work with the plan (pages 237 to 272). Remember that good nutrition plays a crucial role in your energy level and overall health, and it will give you the foundation to keep the pounds off like nothing else. Make smart choices, eat balanced, and stay within the parameters of the program, and you'll be poised for success!

WHAT YOU WILL BE EATING ON THE 7 DAY JUMP START

As we discussed in Chapter 4, the three core components of the 7 Day Jump Start are protein, carbohydrates, and fats. My meals are designed to contain a balance of these three crucial nutrients. If you skipped past that chapter, I encourage you to take a quick look back to get familiar with them.

There's never a reason to sway from the plan—there are always options available to make it work for you. You can swap out any

7 GOALS FOR THE 7 DAY JUMP START

1. Jump start your weight loss
2. Lose up to 5 to 7 pounds quickly
3. Eliminate bloating and water retention
4. Learn healthy "clean eating" habits
5. Naturally eliminate gluten and other processed foods
6. Find a balance of protein, fats, and carbohydrates in your meals
7. Increase your energy and commit to working out

7 DAY JUMP START BASICS

- Eat breakfast. Skipping breakfast means getting overly hungry and overeating later in the day.
- Use your fist as a guide when judging your protein servings (or purchase a food scale).
- Have no more than 2 servings of starchy carbs a day (see page 62 for a list of starches). Aim to get most of your carbs from vegetables and fruits.
- Indulge in as many non-starchy vegetables (steamed or raw) as you like.
- Avoid artificial sweeteners; use stevia as your noncaloric sweetener instead.
- Remove processed cheese from your diet (small amounts of real cheese are OK).
- Don't let yourself get hungry! If you can't get all of the food or meals in a given time, add them to a later meal or have them later in the day.
- Purchase a high-quality protein supplement (see page 60) if you decide to use one.
- Hydrate with 8 to 10 glasses of water a day. Carry water with you, and drink a full glass before your meals.
- Skip the alcohol.
- If you're craving fruit juice, juice whole fruits yourself. Drink one glass and count it as your carb for the meal. Avoid commercial/processed fruit juices.
- Drink your coffee or tea without cream or milk. Add stevia (no other sweeteners) if you need a touch of sweetness.
- Drink as much unsweetened iced or hot green or herbal tea as you like.
- Stock your car/bag/backpack with water, protein, and nuts so you are never without healthy food.
- Keep your snacks and meals to the plan. Look at it this way: 100 calories a day of "nibbles" adds up to about 10 to 12 pounds at the end of the year. So don't "nibble" away at your results!
- Listen to your body. If you are full, stop eating; if you are hungry, eat. Eat all the food in the program; it's up to you if you'd like to break it up between three to six meals.

foods you want, as long as they are in the same category and the same size portion. For instance, instead of chicken, you can have something else, such as fish, from the *protein* list, as long as you keep portion size in mind. If you'd rather eat cucumber than zucchini, go for it! If there are foods you don't like, can't get, or are allergic to, simply swap them out! If you don't care for any particular food, by all means don't force yourself to eat it. There are plenty of delicious healthy swaps to guarantee you'll love every meal you make.

Remember: Protein servings will be 4 to 6 ounces (depending on your sex and size), or the size of your palm or fist (cooked). Starchy carb servings are also about the size of your fist (cooked), which is generally ½ cup cooked, and fats are 1 tablespoon, which will be about the size of your thumb. If you're in that ballpark, you're going to be fine. Steamed or raw vegetables are unlimited!

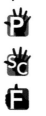

With the exception of these one-for-one swaps, I'm asking you to follow the plan exactly as written for the full seven days, and ideally longer. During this time, even 100 calories worth of nibbles can offset your progress. Remember that it takes seventeen to thirty days to change an old habit and create a new one. This is the critical time when you are turning your habits into your lifestyle! Once you've jump started your weight loss, occasional treat meals are not only allowed but welcomed. Any overly strict weight loss plan is doomed for failure, so always remember the majority rules: If you do what's right most of the time—about 80 percent—and you don't go too crazy on the other 20, you won't have to worry too much about it! That said, if your 20 ends up sabotaging you, then try 90/10 or 95/5. The initial goal is to get you to your ideal goal weight. Once you get there, maintaining is a lot easier than losing.

PROTEIN SWAP-OUTS

The following are examples of your protein choices for the 7 Day Jump Start. Remember, you can always use your hand as a guide to judge portion sizes; it will get you pretty close and works for the long term. A 6′6″ guy will have bigger hands than a 5′1″ woman; serving sizes will reflect that difference, so that's why I give a range of 4 to 6 ounces for protein. And remember that most foods are not all protein, fat, or carb, so some foods might count as more than just a protein.

- 4 to 6 ounces chicken breast
- 4 to 6 ounces dark meat chicken, skinless
- 4 to 6 ounces turkey
- 4- to 6-ounce turkey burger
- 4 to 6 slices turkey breast
- 2 nitrate-free turkey sausages
- 4 to 6 ounces fish (cod, halibut, salmon, tilapia, and any other type)
- About ½ cup shellfish (shrimp, scallops, lobster, crawfish mussels, clams, crab)

4 to 6 ounces lean red meat (beef, lamb, pork, venison; counts as your fat serving, too)

5-ounce can water-packed tuna fish, or another canned fish, such as salmon

2 whole eggs

5 egg whites

1 scoop whey or egg protein powder (see pages 60 to 61 for more on protein powders)

½ cup plain, full-fat Greek yogurt or kefir

½ cup plain, full-fat cottage cheese

½ cup hummus (counts as a carb and a fat, too)

½ cup shelled edamame

THE SCOOP ON PROTEIN SUPPLEMENTS

There are many portable carb and fat sources (think fruit and nuts), but protein is the hardest to have with you at all times, which makes protein powder a quick and convenient way to get an adequate amount of this nutrient. If your meal is light on protein, stir a scoop into a glass of water and just like that, you've made your meal a balanced one.

Protein powder is also a great addition for those of you working out hard; it will help your body grow and repair lean mass, which further boosts your metabolism. But there are so many types of protein powder in a wide range of brands and prices. I personally use several different protein supplements depending on the time of day and how hard I am training. What is most important to me,

is that I am using a protein powder with the least amount of ingredients. Some have a long list of ingredients while others have minimal. With that being said, if I need a quick source of protein on the go, I use whey and egg proteins. For vegans, plant-based protein powders are an option. Whichever you choose, be super careful about avoiding protein powders with added sugars, artificial sweeteners such as aspartame (stevia is OK), and other processed additives. Make sure the label says it's gluten-free (you never know!). For the most part, protein powder should be mixed with water.

Whey Protein Powder

Whey protein is a high-quality protein that is digested very quickly. It is great first thing in the morning, before and after a workout, or when you need to bump up the protein content of a meal. Ideally, use a ½ scoop of whey protein (enough to get 12 to 15 grams of protein) mixed with water, along with a simple piece of fruit such as an apple pre- and post-workout. This gives your muscles the ideal nutrients to get through tough workouts and help your body repair itself afterward. Another huge benefit is that whey helps to control your hunger.

Egg Protein Powder

Egg protein is a slower digesting protein that can be taken anytime, but it is especially good before bed, as it will help your body repair itself while you sleep. This is really important for those people that are working out. Egg protein can be used as part of a meal, or as a meal replacement, and can also be added into baked goods.

Plant-Based Protein Powders

I personally avoid soy protein powders (they are typically extremely processed) in favor of pea, bean, or hemp powders. These are suggested for vegans or those with dairy or egg allergies. If you don't find them as tasty as the other options, try mixing them with almond milk or in a smoothie with some juice or berries.

PROTEIN BARS

Beware: the vast majority of protein bars on the market today are complete junk and have no greater nutritional value than a dollar store candy bar. I understand that if you are a busy person, grabbing fresh foods is not always an option, and if you're looking for a healthy on-the-go snack, a good quality protein bar can be a good option. Be sure to read your label like a sleuth! When you look at a bar and the first three ingredients are soy protein, high-fructose corn syrup, and sugar, you know there's something wrong!

My rule for choosing protein bars is to look for minimally processed bars that are natural, high in protein, gluten-free, and don't contain high-fructose corn syrup or artificial sweeteners. Of course, they also need to taste

great! Read through the ingredients—if you can define them (and you're not a scientist), chances are you are making a decent choice. Protein bars containing raw nuts and seeds, fruit as a sweetener, and quality protein powder (see above) ensure that you will be putting into your body the best foods for energy and recovery from workouts. You might enjoy this short video on my website: www.natalie jillfitness.com/protein-bars/.

FAT SWAP-OUTS

The following are examples of your fat choices for the 7 Day Jump Start. Remember, you can use your thumb to gauge serving sizes.

1 tablespoon unrefined coconut oil, clarified butter, or extra-virgin olive oil

About 8 raw, unsalted nuts

1 tablespoon raw, unsalted pumpkin or sesame seeds

1 tablespoon pine nuts

1 tablespoon no-sugar-added cashew, walnut, or another nut or seed butter

1 tablespoon avocado, approximately

1 hard-boiled egg

1 tablespoon unprocessed cheese

¼ cup hummus

CARBOHYDRATE SWAP OUTS

You get to eat two starchy carbs a day on the Jump Start; the rest of your carbs should come from vegetables and fruits. This means that two meals can contain starchy carbs, and the third will be primarily vegetable- or fruit-based. Remember that vegetables are unlimited, and so are berries. Also, you don't have to have two starchy carbs a day—you are welcome to eat more fruits and vegetables in their place.

Starchy carbs

1 small sweet potato
1 small white potato
½ banana
½ cup gluten-free oatmeal
½ cup cooked quinoa
½ cup cooked brown or white rice
½ cup cooked beans or lentils
½ cup cooked corn
1 slice all-natural gluten-free bread

Non-starchy carbs

1 small orange, grapefruit, pear, or peach
1 cup grapes, melon cubes, or pineapple
1 cup berries (blueberries, raspberries, blackberries, sliced strawberries)
Any vegetable (unlimited; see list below)

VEGETABLES

Vegetables are carbohydrates that are naturally low in calories and full of nutrients that your body needs and craves. Veggies are full of fiber, vitamins, and minerals, which is why I encourage you to eat them abundantly and why they are unlimited on the Jump Start. They add color, texture, and flavor contrast to your plate, and they make a handy on-the-go snack. There's an item on the list that may seem new to you: seaweed. If you think you've never eaten it, you may be surprised to learn that whenever you order sushi, it comes wrapped in seaweed! Seaweed is a powerful antioxidant and an amazing source of minerals, including iodine, critical for healthy thyroid. Seaweed is one of the most nutritious foods around—ounce for ounce it's higher in vitamins and minerals than any other class of food! Today's popular sea snacks make for a crunchy, satisfying between-meal treat, and kids go crazy for them.

Eating plenty of vegetables can help protect you from conditions including arthritis, heart disease, stroke, and cancer, and they'll keep you looking and feeling younger. Listen to this: A recent study found that people who eat seven or more portions of vegetables and fruit a day have over a 40 percent lower risk of dying from any cause compared to those who eat less than one portion, with vegetables having a greater impact than fruit. That's why I've made vegetables unlimited, as long as they are steamed or raw, so feel free to enjoy these freely!

Artichoke hearts (fresh or water packed, jarred)
Artichokes
Asparagus
Bamboo shoots
Beet greens
Bell peppers (any color)
Bok choy

Broccoli	Fennel	Radishes
Brussels sprouts	Garlic	Scallions
Cabbage (red and green)	Jicama	Seaweed
Carrots	Kale	Snow peas
Cauliflower	Kohlrabi	Spinach
Celery	Leeks	Summer squash (yellow)
Chiles	Lettuce	Swiss chard
Cilantro	Mushrooms	Turnip greens
Collard greens	Mustard greens	Watercress
Cucumbers	Okra	Zucchini
Eggplant	Onions	
Endive	Parsley	

FREE FOODS TO SPICE UP YOUR DIET

There are tons of options for pumping up the flavor and nutrition of your food while adding a negligible amount of calories. Think of it this way: if you are eating five or six times a day, that's anywhere from 150 to 180 "meals" per month. It's hard to find that many different foods to eat, so use seasonings to mix it up. Putting together new flavor combinations is where you can get really creative in the kitchen! Here are some easy and tasty options.

Lemon and Lime Juice

Squeeze on some citrus to perk up any plate! Add it to a glass of water (mix in a few drops of stevia for a no-cal lemonade), serve a wedge with your fish, toss it with salad greens, or add it to a marinade for meat.

Lemons and limes are an excellent source of vitamin C, they boost your immune system, help prevent wrinkles, and can even help with weight loss. And they are super detoxifying—squeeze some into hot water first thing in the morning for a clean start to your day!

Cinnamon

Sprinkle a little onto your coffee, oatmeal, or gluten-free toast. It's also delicious paired with root vegetables like carrots or sweet potatoes.

Chiles

There's nothing better to wake up your taste buds than with hot chiles! Choose from milder chiles like jalapeños, cherry peppers, and Spanish pimientos, or opt for a spicier pepper like habanero and Scotch bonnet. If you really like things hot, try the hottest chile on earth, the ghost chile! Chiles contain capsaicin, which is known to relieve pain, support heart health, and stop ulcers. They also can increase endorphin production and metabolism, basically giving you a boost all over! Tabasco sauce can be a nice option; check hot sauce bottle labels and avoid those containing large amounts of sugar and artificial ingredients.

Turmeric

This golden spice is a key ingredient in Indian curries, and its health benefits include anti-inflammatory, antiviral, antibacterial, and antioxidant effects. There's some talk that it's the daily turmeric that's responsible for the significantly lower rates of Alzheimer's disease in India. Add a pinch to any dish to benefit from its amazing health profile; a small amount has little impact on flavor. You can even add it to smoothies and you won't taste it.

Garlic

Just about any savory dish is enhanced by adding garlic. As a bonus, garlic contains antifungal, antibacterial, and antiviral properties. The American Heart Association has acknowledged the benefits of eating garlic, including decreasing blood pressure, blood glucose, and blood pressure.

Herbs

Herbs add variety! Thyme, oregano, rosemary, cilantro, and parsley are just some of the great flavor boosters that go into making a fantastic meal. You won't find fresh herbs in any processed foods, that's for sure! For the freshest herbs, consider growing a window garden so your herbs can go straight from the pot to your plate.

SNACKS

Good snacks ideally will contain healthy fats, protein, and some carbs. The three don't have to appear in the perfect ratio, and you can have a snack with just two of the three, but avoid snacking on pure carbs. Grabbing a piece of fruit? Have about a tablespoon of fat or 3 to 4 ounces of protein with it. The fats and protein are key for keeping you satisfied and stopping cravings and hunger pains in their tracks. Raw green veggies are totally fine to nibble on throughout the day. And keep in mind that snacks aren't mandatory—no need to force-feed yourself if you're not hungry! See pages 125 to 138 for some fantastic snack ideas.

SWEETENERS

You'll be enjoying the following sweeteners in my 7 Day Jump Start dessert recipes (see page 32 for all about unprocessing sugar from your diet):

Fruit
Honey
Maple syrup
Coconut nectar
Agave nectar

DON'T SKIP THE SALT

WE'VE all heard it before: "avoid salt!" But why? Unless you have high blood pressure or are nearing a competition or photo shoot and want to keep any tiny bit of bloat from showing up, eating an adequate amount is a must! In fact, our body needs salt for its very existence.

But when I say that salt is good for you, it's *unrefined* salt I'm talking about. *Refined* white salt, aka table salt, is nutritionally empty, because it has been stripped of the full spectrum of natural minerals. It's an industrially processed product, and there's no place for it in an unprocessed diet.

How to know if a salt is unrefined? Look at the color. Full spectrum salt isn't naturally white, and the more refined it gets, the whiter it gets. While sea salt may be mineral rich, it is often processed to a pearly white color. Look for sea salt that is off-white to gray, or, if your budget allows, Himalayan salt, a pure and unrefined salt option containing large amounts of minerals and trace elements that are easily metabolized by the body.

Here are some of the amazing benefits of unrefined salt:

Losing and maintaining weight: Eating unrefined salt creates digestive juices, which help your body digest and eliminate foods faster.

Feeling good and sleeping tight: Unrefined salt can help preserve melatonin and serotonin, which make you feel good! It also can help you relax, which helps you to sleep better.

Working your muscles: Unrefined salt contains small amounts of potassium, which is critical for helping muscles function properly. And when you sweat, your body loses a lot of sodium. Your body needs salt when you are working out!

Combating cravings: Rather than reaching for highly processed foods to satisfy your cravings, try adding a small amount of unrefined salt to healthy choices like vegetables. You will be surprised by how the salt will satisfy the craving without sacrificing your healthy diet.

So when I ask you to limit or eliminate refined white table salt, it's not because of the extra sodium; it's all about keeping nutritionally empty foods out of your diet! And the next time you hear one of your friends saying that salt is bad for you, you can smile knowing that there are, in fact, many benefits to adding some *unrefined* salt to your nutrition program!

WHAT YOU'LL BE DRINKING ON THE 7 DAY JUMP START

Most of us need to drink more water. On my 7 Day Jump Start, I recommend drinking 8 to 10 glasses of water a day. Water is especially crucial when you are doing any type of exercise. Your body sweats to stay cool, and you lose fluids. This disruption in body fluids can impede your workout if you don't hydrate. I feel more energy when I stay hydrated during a workout.

Hydration means having enough fluid in your body to keep it working properly. Many of us walk around chronically dehydrated without even realizing it. Being dehydrated can cause fatigue, false hunger, irritability, muscle cramps, hormonal swings, GI issues (i.e., constipation), and bloat from chronic water retention. A lot of hunger is actually thirst or dehydration in disguise, so if those hunger pains arise, have a glass of water and see if that doesn't help first. The water will help to resolve any false hunger. If you're still hungry, go ahead and eat; the water will help fill you up so you won't need to eat as much.

The majority of hydration comes from:

- Pure water
- Noncaffeinated beverages (caffeinated beverages provide some hydration, but they are less beneficial because the caffeine acts as a diuretic)
- Foods, and fruits in particular—cantaloupe, cucumber, tomatoes, oranges, grapefruit, and tangerines are among the most hydrating fruits

I hear from a lot of women that bloating is a big issue. They feel bloated, so they stop drinking water, which only makes things worse. By drinking water (and I mean water, not sugar-filled juices or sodas!) consistently throughout the day, your body won't feel the need to retain water. Losing this bloat will make you look and feel better!

It might seem counterintuitive, but to stop bloating, you need to give your body plenty of fluids so it doesn't feel the need to retain water. Staying hydrated speeds up your metabolism, will keep you feeling energized and awake, allows your body to feel and function much better, and you'll be able better to ascertain whether you're truly hungry or slightly dehydrated.

KEEPING TRACK OF YOUR HYDRATION

- Always have a clean reusable water bottle or packs of disposable water bottles available. Keep one in your home, your car, on your bicycle, at work, and at the gym.
- Keep track of your ounces' intake (the notes feature on your smartphone is a good way specifically to track hydration).
- If you carry a daily water bottle, figure out how much yours holds, and keep your water intake on track!

SHOULD YOU ADD SUPPLEMENTS?

Before we start talking about supplements, I want to be clear about something: supplements are called *supplements* for a reason. If they were anything more, they would be called *fundamentals*. Your overall lifestyle, nutrition, and the food you eat are fundamental to being healthy. Many people want to skip the fundamentals and jump straight to supplements. The problem is, there is no supplement out there that will do more for you than any fundamental. That means that you have to have your fundamentals down—drinking

DRINKING YOUR CALORIES IS A WASTE

SODAS and sports drinks are a giant source of calories that hold little to no nutritional value. You're simply filling your body up with artificial chemicals that do absolutely nothing for your body. What a waste! Those calories add up quickly and you've got nothing to show for it.

On my plan, you don't need to drink juices or sugary sports drinks to stay hydrated. Instead, focus on making sure you're fully hydrated by drinking water, unsweetened teas, and moderate amounts of fresh-pressed organic juices. If you're involved in an extended period of cardiovascular activity (such as a run of ninety minutes or more), or it's especially hot and you're sweating a lot, then you can consider a "sports drink" or electrolyte replacement mix, just keep an eye on the sugar content. Most people overestimate their need for "sports drinks" when exercising. You shouldn't need a hyped-up "sports drink" for a regular workout that's less than 90 minutes. Most of the time, water is all that's needed.

enough water, eating balanced meals, moving, and so on. You can't skip the fundamentals, fill yourself with junk, and expect the latest and greatest weight-loss supplement to make up for that, no matter what the ad says. Make sure you have a healthy lifestyle so you are more likely to experience the benefits of those supplements.

That said, supplements can and do have a place for many people. For example, if your body is deficient in a certain vitamin or mineral and your doctor says you need to supplement with "Vitamin X" or "Mineral Y" to be healthy, that's perfectly fine. What I'm mostly focusing on here are the weight-loss and diet supplements that run in ads and infomercials nonstop on TV, in magazines, and on the radio. Just because you are bombarded with "take this pill and lose weight" day after day doesn't make it true. The same is true for the guys who are usually targeted with "easy" ways to pack on muscle quickly with little effort (which we know doesn't happen).

In addition to the weight-loss pills, there are so many supplement choices, so many products, and sometimes less than knowledgeable salespeople telling you why you should buy something. The wrong information may not only put a very large dent in your pocketbook; it can give you false hope and disappointment, and even make you sick.

I do, however, believe many supplements can have a place but for the right reasons. Keep in mind that there are no magic pills. There isn't a pill or drink that will make you leaner or stronger.

When shopping for supplements, look for brands with a high standard of product quality. I look for pure-sourced ingredients and companies that value sustainability for not only us, but for the planet. I look at research and quality control, and I make sure everything is tested. The supplements I recommend are a good multivitamin, green powder, fish oil, B vitamins, and magnesium.

MULTIVITAMINS

A good multivitamin is like an insurance plan. Most of your nutrition should come through proper nutrition, but a high-quality vitamin supplement can be good insurance. If your body does not use the vitamins, the excess will merely be excreted. If your doctor has run the proper blood tests and tells you that you are deficient in a specific vitamin, then definitely supplement with that vitamin.

GREEN POWDER

Even if you are eating enough vegetables, it can still be very hard to eat a good amount of leafy greens each and every day. Supplementing with a concentrated greens supplement is a convenient way of consistently getting in your greens. The benefits range from boosting your energy levels, to helping digestion, and purifying and enhancing your immune system. Follow the recommended amounts on the label.

FISH OIL

Fish oil is important to the body because it contains omega-3 fatty acids. These fatty acids are important for heart and cardiovascular health, they help combat depression and arthritis, and have great anti-inflammatory properties. The two main omega-3 fatty acids are DHA (docosahexaenoic acid) and EPA (eicosapentaenoic acid), so make sure your fish oil supplement has both, and in high amounts. Shoot for at least 1000 milligrams of fish oil per day, which is typically one to two capsules depending on the brand. Vegetarians can swap in flax oil, but know that it's not as powerful a source, as its omega-3 profile comes from ALA (alpha-linolenic acid), which must then be converted to EPA/DHA. The conversion is fairly inefficient, with the result less usable EPA/DHA in flax oil.

B VITAMINS

There are several B vitamins, and they are commonly combined into a B-vitamin supplement, although they can be found individually as well. In a nutshell, B vitamins help the body get and make energy from the food you eat. In addition, they also help form red blood cells. B vitamins are commonly found in meat, dairy, and leafy greens.

B vitamins are all water-soluble, so any excess is easily removed from the body.

MAGNESIUM

Magnesium is a favorite supplement of mine for calming me at night and helping me sleep. In addition, it helps to keep you regular, and it really helps keep those PMS symptoms and cravings in check, at least for me anyway.

Remember, supplements are meant to *supplement* your diet and hard work. They are not meant to *replace* it. No supplement can take the place of a fundamental!

Note: You'll want to check with your health-care professional before starting any supplements; there may be contraindications with supplements and medications you may be taking.

WHAT YOU *WON'T* BE EATING OR DRINKING ON THE 7 DAY JUMP START

- Processed foods
- Ingredients you can't pronounce or define
- Any meal in a box or a plastic tray
- Gluten-containing foods (wheat, rye, barley, triticale)
- Processed soy
- High-fructose corn syrup and table sugar
- Artificial sweeteners
- Trans fats
- Processed junk cheese
- Cream or sweetener in your coffee/tea
- Alcohol (you can do it for seven days— be the designated driver at every event!)
- Fruit juice (unless you're juicing whole fruits yourself, in which case you can have 1 glass a day—count it as your carb)

I know what you're thinking—that's a pretty short list, isn't it? That's right—for the next seven days you'll be eating abundantly delicious, real foods while remembering to avoid these few foods. You've got this!

PRACTICING MINDFUL EATING

Have you ever been sitting in front of the television, talking on the phone, or even driving in the car, and you weren't even aware of what or how much you've eaten?

You look down and suddenly there's an empty plate or food container, and you don't even remember enjoying it. Not only that, but you're still hungry! I call this eating on autopilot, or "unconscious eating." The reason you're still hungry is because you haven't been conscious of your activities, and you haven't allowed your brain to process the fullness cues that let you know when to stop eating.

I know you're busy and sometimes have to fit in meals while completing other tasks, but for these seven days, I want you to find the time and focus on your food whenever possible. That means eliminating eating on autopilot and, instead, practicing mindful eating.

Mindful eating means:

- No eating in front of the television
- No eating at your desk while on your computer
- No eating in the car (except for an emergency 6 to 8 nuts when you're stuck in traffic)
- No eating standing up at your kitchen counter or anywhere else

Instead, I'd like you to make your meal, sit down at a table, and think about each bite. Be conscious of slowing your pace, chewing every bite, and letting your body do its thing. Chewing is where digestion starts, so don't "inhale" your meal if you are in a rush. Take an extra minute or two to enjoy it, and listen to your body for those cues for fullness. Keeping yourself accountable for what you eat is an important key to weight-loss success. As a bonus, you'll have a newfound appreciation for your food!

USING MANTRAS TO FOCUS YOUR MIND

THINK of an energizing statement that puts you into a motivated state of mind. Find a mantra you can repeat to help drive out negative energy and remind you of your goals. You can use your vision board (page 25) for your inspiration.

Some mantras that I've used:

- I love myself for everything I am.
- I am ready to be my best me.
- I am happy, healthy, and fit.
- I've got this!

15 REASONS WHY THE 7 DAY JUMP START WILL WORK FOR YOU

1. It is about addition, not subtraction (or deprivation)
2. It teaches you how to make the right food choices
3. You can implement these simple changes anywhere on any budget
4. It is empowering, not discouraging
5. You get immediate results—more energy and feeling better all around!
6. Bloat and fatigue go away
7. You will lose fat
8. It is safe for your whole family
9. It is based on real food, not "diet" food or fake processed foods or supplements
10. It is common sense
11. It is easy
12. The food tastes great
13. You won't be hungry
14. It keeps you accountable
15. You'll feel so great you'll want to make it a lifestyle

DAVID'S TRANSFORMATION:

From an ineffective diet to a "second nature"
way of eating—and minus 20 pounds and 4 inches of belly fat!

Processed foods = low energy and back pain: Before the Jump Start, my diet consisted of beer, pizza, cheeseburgers, and basically anything I felt like eating. I felt bloated, had low energy, and was uncomfortable with my weight. I ate out often and never paid attention to what I was getting and whether or not it was healthy. I would eat/snack on the couch in front of the TV. I sat often (watching TV or working at my desk) and my back would always hurt. When I was trying to eat healthy, I was grabbing the wrong foods with misleading labels. I knew I wasn't feeling great but when I got married and saw how I looked in the photos, I knew I had to do something.

A chance meeting: I would go to the gym and use machines and weights. I was bored with my usual routine and didn't feel like it was changing my body much. I felt like I was just going through the motions and became discouraged which led to me eating even more comfort foods. Then I discovered Natalie Jill through work—I'm a videographer and I work with Natalie on her YouTube videos. I learned about Natalie's Jump Start lifestyle plan while filming with her over the last few years. I'd heard about unprocessed eating but wasn't sure how to go about it—eating an unprocessed diet seemed like a lot of work. And there in front of me, literally, was someone telling me how to do it!

The Jump Start becomes second nature: It turns out that Jump Start is very doable. With Jump Start it is easier to consistently eat healthy because I learned the proper ratios to be eating at each meal. It eventually becomes second nature to look for the better options using the ratios when eating out and grocery shopping. Plus all the snack options kept me satisfied and not feeling hungry. It's even OK to slip up sometimes—if you do just go back to the program again and you'll get yourself back on track.

I eat a lot of vegetables with every meal. I eat lean protein like fish, turkey, and chicken. If I drink alcohol, it's consciously and only occasionally. I routinely change up the types of vegetables I eat and try to mix up the proteins at every meal. This helps keep it fresh. I prep all of my meals ahead of time so it is easier to make healthy foods during the week when I am busy. I can make healthy meals on the fly because I only keep healthy options at home and know the protein/carb/fat ratios so it's VERY easy. I do not eat out as much as I used to, but when I do, I eat a healthy snack beforehand so I don't go hungry and this allows me to make a better, healthier decision when it comes to choosing what I order. I only eat at the kitchen table. I now use a stand-up desk and exercise regularly. Using bodyweight exercises allows me to work out at home and fits into my busy schedule.

Lose the bloat and the pain—gain energy and confidence: I lost more than 20 pounds and 4 inches off my waist. I'm not bloated and uncomfortable anymore. I no longer have back pain now that I am strengthening my core and building muscle. Eating healthy and making healthier choices is now so easy. I couldn't imagine going back to how I was eating before. This has become a lifestyle. I feel great and am loving the results.

DAVID BEFORE   DAVID AFTER

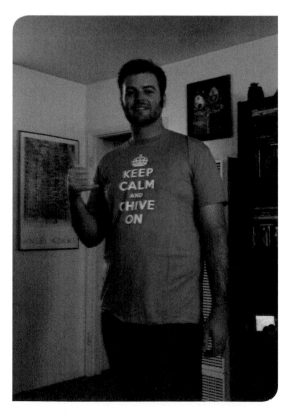

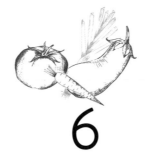

6

SHOPPING FOR THE 7 DAY JUMP START

"Be smart when you fill up your cart!"

YOU can find most of the wholesome ingredients on the Jump Start right in your grocery store. I'll talk more about organics and non-GMO foods in a minute, but for the best organic selection, make a visit to your neighborhood natural foods store or co-op. And if you want to get really excited about seasonal fruits and veggies, get acquainted with your local farmers' market. The website www.localharvest.org will help you locate the market nearest to you. Grocery shopping can be quick, easy, and fun if you know what to look for. Here are some guidelines to take the stress out of shopping:

Do *not* go to the grocery store hungry. Grocery shopping and a hungry belly is a bad combination. Grocery shopping hungry will cloud your decision-making, as cravings start to kick in and willpower gets left in the car. If you can't avoid shopping on a hungry belly, pop some almonds or cashews in your mouth and drink some water to stave off the hunger and keep you from impulse buying.

Shop the store perimeter. The outside perimeter of the store is where you'll find real food. This is where the fresh stuff— fruits, veggies, meats, and seafood—are typically located. Visit them frequently to pick up your weekly staples, with jaunts into the aisles for other unprocessed foods such as nuts and whole grains. You will notice that the inside of the grocery store is lined with processed and packaged foods. This is where you will find rows and rows of cans, boxes, and bags of food. This is *not* what we want to be eating.

Read labels. If you do not know what something on the label means, it is likely very processed and you should consider putting it back. The closer to the natural state a food once was, the better it is for you. Think land, sea, ground, and tree. A good basic rule is that if an item has more than five ingredients, you probably don't want it in your cart—or in your stomach.

Don't buy something just because it says it's gluten-free. For the most part, real foods won't have labels or stickers on them. But don't be fooled by processed foods just because they have "gluten-free" stamped on them. Do your research, read labels, and choose a grocery store that generally has more natural foods and minimally processed options. My favorite meal-replacement bars and shakes are minimally processed. So are quinoa and brown rice. But remember: just because a label trumpets "gluten-free" doesn't mean that it's any better for you than anything else. In some cases, it can even be worse for weight loss! Stick with naturally gluten-free foods—the ones on the perimeter rather than in the aisles—instead of processed foods.

Buy in bulk. Bulk purchases can save you two of our most important commodities: money and time. Get to know stores that deal in large quantities, including the freezer and produce sections. Stock your freezer with fish, chicken, veggies, and even frozen berries, and instantly you will have access to easy-to-make meals. You can find lots of items in bulk online as well. You can learn about another great option for saving money on groceries here: www.nataliejillfitness.com /thrive-market.

Choose an ideal time. Pick a day and time of the week that is slower for you and do your shopping then; then when you come home, immediately prepare a few meals and store them in your fridge or freeze them. This way you will have your food at the ready to reheat when you're hungry.

YOUR UNPROCESSED LIFESTYLE SHOPPING LIST

This list includes everything you'll need to follow the basic 7 Day Jump Start menu plan. (This list does not include the swap-out options or the recipe options.)

So when you're ready to start your 7 Day Jump Start, fill your kitchen with foods from the list below and supplement with choices from any individual Jump Start recipe that you'd like to use in place of the basic meal plan. At the end of the Basic 7 Day Jump Start list, I'll share with you my full everyday, unprocessed pantry list to take you beyond the seven days to an eating plan for a lifetime.

And remember that you can swap out ingredients as you like according to the guidelines on page 95. Now you're ready to unprocess your diet for week one and more! Who wants some?

FOR THE BASIC 7 DAY JUMP START PLAN

Meat, Poultry, and Fish

Whenever possible, choose: wild over farmed for fish, and nitrate-free, free-range, and organic for meat

Chicken breast   Scallops

Chicken thighs   Shrimp

Turkey bacon

Turkey breast

Turkey sausage

Ground turkey

Fresh salmon

Smoked salmon

Fresh tuna

Halibut

Extra proteins

Edamame

Hummus

Dairy, Eggs, and Butter

Choose full fat for dairy and cage-free and organic for eggs whenever possible

Plain Greek yogurt

Goat cheese

Cottage cheese

Feta cheese

Eggs

Butter

Ghee

Fresh Herbs and Seasonings

Basil

Capers

Cilantro

Ginger

Starchy Vegetables

Sweet potatoes

Non-Starchy Vegetables

Bell peppers   Red onion

Bok choy   Salad mix

Carrots   Sliced mushrooms

Celery   Spinach

Cucumbers   Sugar snap peas

Garlic   Swiss chard

Kale   Yellow onion

Lettuce   Zucchini

Napa cabbage

Portobello mushrooms

Fruits

Apples   Melon

Avocado   Mixed berries

Bananas   Oranges

Cherry tomatoes Peaches

Grapes   Pears

Lemons   Raspberries

Limes   Strawberries

Mango   Tomatoes

PANTRY INGREDIENTS

Oils	*Grains*	*Nuts and Seeds*
Coconut oil Extra-virgin olive oil	Oatmeal	Almonds Macadamia nuts Walnuts Pine nuts Sesame seeds

Dried Spices and Flavorings	*Boxed, Bottled, and Canned Foods*

Black pepper   Himalayan salt or
Cinnamon   unrefined sea salt
	Balsamic vinegar Red wine vinegar
	Gluten-free seeded Sun-dried tomatoes
	    crackers Whey protein
	No-sugar-added powder
	    almond butter

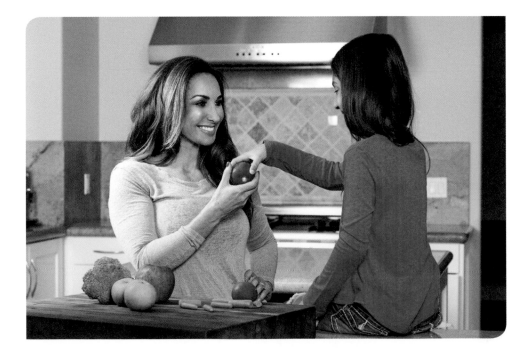

YOUR FULLY STOCKED UNPROCESSED PANTRY
(FOR THE SEVEN DAYS AND BEYOND)

Oils

Coconut oil (unrefined or virgin)

Extra-virgin olive oil

Extra-virgin olive oil cooking spray

Toasted sesame oil

Starchy Carbs/Grains and Beans

Brown or white rice

Rice noodles

All-natural gluten-free bread

Lentils/beans

Quinoa or another gluten-free whole grain

Rolled oats

Nuts and Seeds

Almond butter (no-sugar-added) or another nut butter

Almonds

Cashews

Macadamia nuts

Pecans

Pine nuts

Pistachios

Walnuts

Chia seeds

Flax seeds

Hemp seeds

Pumpkin seeds

Sesame seeds

Shredded coconut

Coconut flakes

Flours and Baking Ingredients

Almond flour

Coconut flour

Tapioca flour

Gluten-free oat flour

Gluten-free oat bran

Cocoa powder

Cacao nibs

Dark chocolate

Baking soda

Baking powder

Dried Spices and Flavorings

Himalayan salt or unrefined sea salt

Black pepper

Cinnamon

Nutmeg

Allspice

Pumpkin pie spice

Bay leaves

Cayenne

Chili powder

Crushed red pepper

Cumin powder

Curry powder

Garlic powder

Garlic salt

Onion powder

Oregano

Paprika

Parsley

Rosemary

Thyme

Almond extract

Vanilla extract

YOUR FULLY STOCKED UNPROCESSED PANTRY *continued*

Sweeteners

Agave nectar	Coconut sugar	Maple syrup
Coconut nectar	Honey	

Dry Goods, Bottled and Canned Foods

Coconut milk	Canned artichoke hearts	Gluten-free tamari sauce
Canned chickpeas	Sun-dried tomatoes	Mustard
Almond milk (unsweetened)	Thai chile paste	Vegetable stock
Balsamic vinegar	Olives	Chicken stock
Apple cider vinegar	Capers	Protein powder (optional)
Red wine vinegar	Sriracha sauce	
Rice vinegar	Wasabi paste	Gluten-free crackers
White wine vinegar	Coconut aminos (available in natural food stores, often found on the shelf with another alternative to soy sauce, gluten-free tamari sauce)	
Red cooking wine		
Tomato juice		
Canned tomatoes		
Tomato paste		

GOING ORGANIC

Is organic worth the extra cost? I personally feel it is for my family. Here are some of the reasons why:

No toxins: Would you rather eat food that had chemicals and pesticides all over it, or one that didn't? I know it isn't always practical or affordable to eat everything organic, but there are some foods that it is most important to eat organic. I have included a list of twelve foods you should try to get organic when you can. (See page 80.)

No GMOs: The use of GMOs (genetically modified organisms) is not permitted during any stage of organic food production or processing.

Heart healthy: Organic milk and meat are typically higher in CLA (conjugated linoleic acid) and omega-3 fatty acids, two heart-healthy fats that can improve our health.

Pesticide-free: Over one billion pounds of pesticides are used in the United States each year on our crops. We then consume some of these chemicals as pesticide residue on fruits and vegetables. When we eat organic, we are eating pesticide-free.

Healthy pregnancy and baby: During pregnancy, the chemicals we eat will reach your baby through the umbilical cord and will be passed through your breast milk if you breastfeed. Please, feed your baby organic baby food. You want baby's first foods to be the purest possible!

Child friendly: Organic food diets in children greatly reduce pesticide exposure, which can lower pesticide levels in children's bodies.

Better taste: You can taste the difference in organic food. Don't believe me? Do a taste test yourself! Purchase some organic and nonorganic berries. Close your eyes and taste them. I'd be surprised if you didn't taste a difference.

Better for the animals: Raising organic livestock means that they are fed good nutrition, which ultimately keeps them healthy, strong, and productive. They are given humane living conditions and not given antibiotics or injections of growth hormones, which ultimately we consume.

How do you know if what you are eating is organic?

Grow it yourself, buy local, or get smart about reading the labels. In the stores, foods must meet the USDA organic standard to wear this label. If it is not, it likely is not organic.

Farmers' markets are popping up all over the place. Check www.localharvest.org to find one in your area. Look for market stalls that sell organic produce, dairy, and meat.

There are several classifications of organic:

100% Organic: Products that are completely organic or made with all organic ingredients

Organic: Products that are at least 95 percent organic

"Made with organic ingredients": Products with at least 70 percent organic ingredients, but can't wear the organic seal

"Natural": Does *not* mean organic. It's more of a marketing term, so don't be fooled!

Note that some small farmers do not have organic certification (it is expensive)—but that doesn't mean they use pesticides. If you're at the farmers' market and aren't sure, ask!

What if you can't buy organic all the time?

Do what you can to start and at least stay away from the "Dirty Dozen," foods that, according to the Environmental Working Group, are best purchased organic, as their conventionally grown counterparts are shown to retain

the highest amounts of harmful chemicals.
The list is ranked in order of worst offenders.

Apples	Celery	Snap peas (imported)
Peaches	Spinach	Potatoes
Nectarines	Sweet bell peppers	Plus these add-ons: hot
Strawberries	Cucumbers	peppers, kale, and collard
Grapes	Cherry tomatoes	greens

WHAT ARE GMOs?

SCIENTISTS now have the ability to insert antifungal, antiviral, and toxic insecticide elements into foods at the genetic level. So foods that contain genetically modified organisms (GMOs) have insecticides *inside* the crop instead of sprayed outside of the crop. And technically, you the consumer are eating those pesticides, too! More than 80 percent of corn and more than 90 percent of soybeans grown in the United States are genetically modified. Canola and cotton-seed oil and their by-products are common GMO foods, and GMO crops are added to processed foods as oils, sweeteners, soy protein, and much more. If you're concerned about keeping GMOs out of your diet, the only way to avoid them is to eat organic. By law, organic products must not contain GMOs.

Because GMOs are relatively new—they first hit grocery store shelves in 1996—there are no long-term studies of the health hazards. But recently the World Health Organization has classified glyphosate, a weed killer routinely sprayed on genetically modified crops, as possibly causing cancer. Since the foods are not labeled (though there is now a strong movement pushing for labeling), there isn't a direct way to link the food sources with health issues. Look for products with the "Non-GMO Project Verified" seal to stay GMO-free.

THE CORN AND SOY QUESTION

ALTHOUGH corn in its grain form does not contain gluten, it can cause some of the same problems for some people. Many celiacs in particular have an intolerance to corn, so it makes a lousy substitute for wheat. Corn has a high starch content, which means it is an inflammatory food, and inflammation has been linked to a whole host of degenerative diseases, including arthritis and cancer. Plus, more than 80 percent of the US corn crops are genetically modified. If a summer barbecue just doesn't make sense to you without corn on the cob, enjoy a small ear and count it as your carb for the meal.

When it comes to soy, the Asian diets are often cited, as soy products have been eaten in Asia for thousands of years. A more accurate reason the Asian diets are healthier may be due to the large consumption of fruits, vegetables, and fish as compared to Western cultures and the *type* of soy they enjoy (see below).

Soy contains a substance called phytoestrogen (aka isoflavones), which mimics natural estrogen. Soybeans contain two types of isoflavones: daidzein and genistein. These compounds are part of a larger group of chemicals called flavonoids that are common in many of the fruits, vegetables, and legumes we eat. But soybeans are the most concentrated form of isoflavones that we get in our diets, which means soy products can potentially raise our estrogen levels and have a negative effect on our health. If you're taking medications or supplements for health conditions such as menopause or breast or ovarian cancer, consult your doctor about minimizing or removing soy from your diet.

There are mixed viewpoints on the effects of consuming soy. Possible positive effects: it may reduce heart disease, help menopause symptoms, treat and prevent osteoporosis, and reduce or prevent some forms of cancer. On the negative side: it may cause hypothyroidism, and fertility issues in women, and it may aggravate gout. One thing I know for sure about soy is that it's big business. In the US alone, we consume in excess of $4 billion in soy products each year, and at this point soy lobbies are equal in number and size to meat and dairy lobbies.

One important reason to avoid soy is that most of the US supply—more than 90 percent—is genetically modified (see page 80 for more on GMOs). If you do include soy in your diet, at a minimum avoid overly processed soy products such as soy milk, soy cheese, soy yogurt, soy butter, and meat substitutes, as well as soy by-products including hydrolyzed soy protein, soy protein isolates, defatted soy flour, textured vegetable protein, soy concentrates, and soy protein concentrates—these act as fillers in many processed food products.

Seek out organic soy options and favor the purest, least processed forms of soy—the ones that are enjoyed in those healthy Asian diets I mentioned above. These include edamame (fresh soybeans—often found in the pod on Japanese restaurant menus), natto (fermented soybeans), miso (fermented soybean paste), and tempeh (soybeans fermented into a cake).

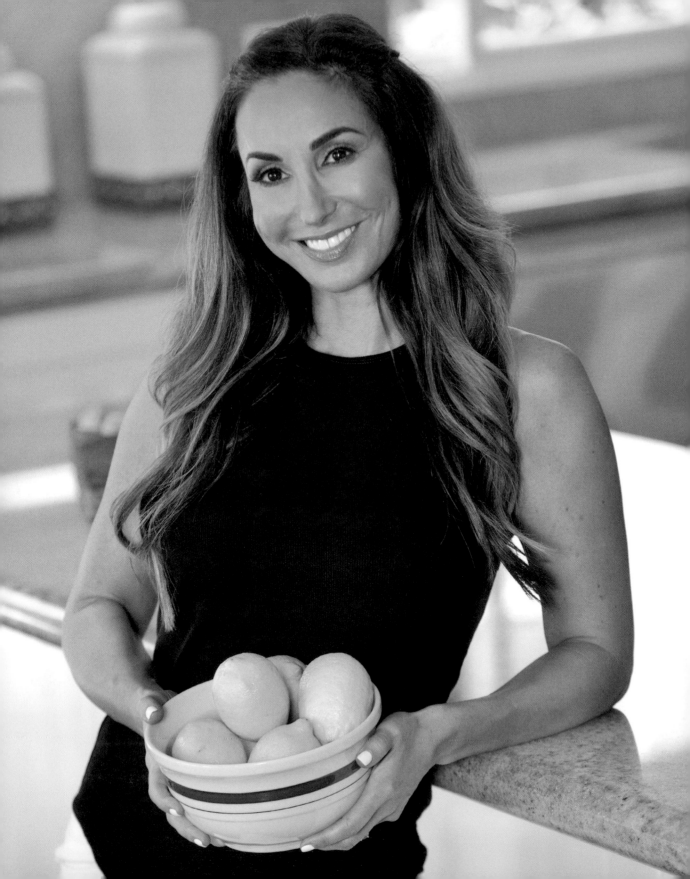

7

BUILDING YOUR UNPROCESSED MEALS— INCLUDING YOUR 7 DAY MEAL PLAN

"Think addition, not subtraction."

NOW'S the time to put together all that you've learned about unprocessing your diet and take it into the kitchen! We've stocked your kitchen with everything you need to complete the Jump Start, so now we can dive right into building your meals for each of the seven days. We'll finish with handy tips on eating out, making a meal out of limited options, being vegetarian on the Jump Start, and what to do when hunger and cravings hit.

If you haven't yet read through Chapter 5: What You'll Be Eating on the 7 Day Jump Start—The Guidelines, I'd like you to flip back and get acquainted with the specifics. The key to the plan is portion control, keeping it simple, and remembering that most of

your meals will contain a balance of protein, carbohydrates, and fats.

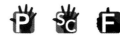

- Protein servings are about the size of your palm or fist, or 4 to 6 ounces for poultry and fish (4 ounces for red meat), or ½ cup beans.
- Starchy carb servings are about ½ cup for whole grains, a small sweet potato, or a small fruit.
- Starchy carbs should be part of up to two of your meals, with non-starchy carbs as part of the third meal.
- Vegetables are unlimited (as long as they are steamed or raw). Potatoes and

corn are considered a starch rather than a vegetable.

- A fat serving is 1 tablespoon fat, about 8 nuts, or 1 tablespoon avocado (about the size of your thumb is a good guideline).
- Dairy should be full-fat.

- Sweeteners include fruit, honey, agave nectar, coconut nectar, and maple syrup.

See pages 59–62 for a list of swap-out options for proteins, carbs, and fat.

7 DAY MEAL PLANS

DAY 1

BREAKFAST

Scrambled Eggs with Berries
1 tablespoon coconut oil (for cooking eggs)
2 eggs, beaten (or swap in 1 nitrate-free turkey sausage or 2 slices nitrate-free turkey bacon)
Himalayan salt or unrefined salt and freshly ground black pepper
1 cup mixed berries

INSTRUCTIONS: Heat the oil in a skillet over medium heat. Add the eggs and scramble to your liking; season with salt and pepper. Serve with the berries.

or

JUMP START RECIPE OPTION: Crab, Spinach, and Mushroom Omelet (page 120)

SNACK
Small piece of fruit (such as an apple, orange, peach, pear, or ½ banana)
1 tablespoon no-sugar-added almond butter

LUNCH

Chicken salad made with the following:
½ cup shredded chicken (or swap in nitrate-free turkey, grilled fish, or shrimp)
2 cups shredded romaine lettuce
1 cup sliced raw vegetables of choice (such as bell peppers and cucumbers)
½ cup julienned cucumber
Himalayan salt and freshly ground black pepper to taste
1 tablespoon extra-virgin olive oil
Juice of ½ lemon

or

JUMP START RECIPE OPTION: Asian Salad (page 141)

SNACK

1 hard-boiled egg
1 tablespoon hummus
2 celery stalks, ½ sliced cucumber, and
    1 sliced green or red bell pepper

or

3 ounces smoked salmon
1 sliced cucumber
¼ cup sliced red onion
½ tablespoon goat cheese
1 teaspoon capers

DINNER

Chicken Thighs with Sweet Potato and Greens

1 to 2 chicken thighs
Himalayan salt and freshly ground black
    pepper to taste
2 cups salad mix
2 teaspoons olive oil
1 teaspoon balsamic vinegar
½ sweet potato
1 teaspoon coconut oil, melted
Ground cinnamon (optional)

INSTRUCTIONS: Season the chicken thighs with salt and pepper and grill, bake, or broil them. Toss the salad mix with the olive oil and vinegar and place on a plate. Top with the chicken and sweet potato, drizzle with the coconut oil, and sprinkle with cinnamon if you like.

or

JUMP START RECIPE OPTION: Cilantro Lime Drumsticks (page 189) and Sweet Potato "Fries" (page 169)

DAY 2

BREAKFAST

Spinach and Goat Cheese Scramble

1 teaspoon extra-virgin olive oil or ghee
    (for cooking eggs)
2 eggs, beaten (or swap in 1 nitrate-free
    turkey sausage or 2 slices nitrate-free
    turkey bacon)
½ cup spinach leaves
1 tablespoon chopped tomatoes
Himalayan salt and freshly ground black
    pepper to taste
1 tablespoon goat cheese

INSTRUCTIONS: Heat the oil in a skillet over medium heat. Add the eggs, spinach, and tomatoes and scramble to your liking; season with salt and pepper. Top with the goat cheese.

or

JUMP START RECIPE OPTION: Egg Muffin (page 117)

SNACK

2 celery stalks
1 tablespoon no-sugar-added
    almond butter

or

JUMP START RECIPE OPTION: 4 Hummus Deviled Egg (page 129) halves

LUNCH

Seared Tuna with Napa Cabbage

1 head Napa cabbage, shredded with
    mixed leaf lettuce
Lemon juice to taste
Himalayan salt and freshly ground black
    pepper to taste
6 ounces tuna, seared
½ cup shelled, cooked edamame
¼ avocado, thinly sliced
1 teaspoon sesame seeds

INSTRUCTIONS: Place the cabbage on a plate and toss with lemon juice; season with salt and pepper. Top with the tuna, edamame, and avocado and sprinkle with the sesame seeds.

or

JUMP START RECIPE OPTION: Seared Tuna Salad (page 143)

SNACK

8 almonds
Small piece of fruit (such as an apple,
    orange, peach, pear, or ½ banana)

DINNER

Shrimp with Bok Choy and Kale

1 tablespoon coconut oil
1 cup chopped bok choy
1 cup chopped kale leaves
6 ounces shrimp (or swap in scallops, white
    fish, or chicken)
Himalayan salt and freshly ground black
    pepper to taste

INSTRUCTIONS: Heat the oil in a skillet over medium heat. Add the bok choy and kale and sauté until wilted. Add the shrimp and cook, tossing, until the shrimp turns opaque. Season with salt and pepper.

or

JUMP START RECIPE OPTION: Garlic Shrimp (page 210) and (Grilled Asparagus on page 163)

DAY 3

BREAKFAST

Option 1: Zucchini Scramble

1 teaspoon butter or ghee
(for cooking eggs)
1 large zucchini, shredded or grated and
squeezed of excess water
2 eggs, beaten (or swap in 1 nitrate-free
turkey sausage or 2 slices nitrate-free
turkey bacon)
½ cup cherry tomatoes, cut in half
Himalayan salt and freshly ground black
pepper to taste
¼ avocado, sliced

INSTRUCTIONS: Heat the butter in a skillet over medium heat. Add the zucchini and cook until softened. Add the eggs and scramble to your liking. Add the cherry tomatoes and stir until softened. Season with salt and pepper and top with the avocado.

Option 2: Smoothie

½ cup frozen mixed berries
½ frozen banana
1 tablespoon unsweetened nut butter
of choice
Juice of 1 orange
1 scoop natural vanilla whey protein
powder *or* ½ cup plain Greek yogurt
½ cup water

INSTRUCTIONS: Combine all the ingredients in a blender and blend until smooth.

or

JUMP START RECIPE OPTION: Crustless Quiche (page 124)

SNACK

1 tablespoon hummus
1 sliced bell pepper and 1 sliced cucumber

or

JUMP START RECIPE OPTION: Figs and Ricotta (page 127)

LUNCH

Basil Chicken

1 teaspoon coconut oil
6 ounces chicken breast (or swap in
nitrate-free turkey breast or grilled fish)
Himalayan salt or unrefined salt and
freshly ground black pepper
1 cup lettuce
1 cup chopped vegetables
Leaves of 4 sprigs of basil, chopped
1 teaspoon extra-virgin olive oil
1 teaspoon balsamic vinegar
1 teaspoon pine nuts

INSTRUCTIONS: Heat the coconut oil in a skillet over medium heat. Season the chicken breast with salt and pepper and cook on both sides until cooked through. In a bowl, combine the lettuce, chopped vegetables, and basil. Season with salt and pepper and toss with the olive oil and vinegar. Top with the chicken and pine nuts.

or

JUMP START RECIPE OPTION: Chicken Avocado Soup (page 153)

SNACK

½ cup plain Greek yogurt
½ cup berries
1 tablespoon sliced almonds

INSTRUCTIONS: Mix the ingredients together to make a parfait.

or

JUMP START RECIPE OPTION: Hummus Deviled Eggs (page 129)

DINNER

1 tablespoon coconut or extra-virgin olive oil

1 teaspoon minced ginger
1 to 2 cloves garlic, diced
½ yellow onion, sliced
2 cups Swiss chard or bok choy
6 ounces sea scallops (or swap in shrimp, white fish, or chicken)
Himalayan salt or unrefined salt and freshly ground black pepper

INSTRUCTIONS: Heat the oil in a skillet over medium heat. Add the ginger, garlic, and onion and sauté until the onion is translucent. Add the Swiss chard or bok choy and cook until wilted. Season the scallops with salt and pepper and cook until opaque on both sides.

or

JUMP START RECIPE OPTION: Pan Seared Scallops with Lemon Vinaigrette (page 209)

DAY 4

BREAKFAST

¼ cup plain Greek yogurt
½ banana, sliced
½ cup raspberries
1 tablespoon chopped almonds

INSTRUCTIONS: Pour the yogurt into a bowl and top with the banana, raspberries, and almonds.

or

JUMP START RECIPE OPTION: Raspberry Twist Smoothie (page 105)

SNACK

½ cup cottage cheese
½ cup red or green grapes
6 sliced almonds
Cinnamon for sprinkling

or

JUMP START RECIPE OPTION: 1 cup Chicken and Kale Soup (page 154) topped with 1 tablespoon Lime Guacamole (page 157)

LUNCH
Turkey and Mixed Vegetables
1 cup mixed vegetables
1 teaspoon coconut oil
6 ounces ground turkey (or swap in thinly sliced chicken breast)
Juice of ½ lime
Himalayan salt or unrefined sea salt and freshly ground black pepper
1 tablespoon feta cheese or ¼ avocado

INSTRUCTIONS: Place the mixed veggies on a plate. Heat the turkey with the oil in a skillet over medium heat until the turkey is cooked through. Drain if necessary, season with salt and pepper, and add to the plate over the vegetables. Top with lime juice and feta cheese or avocado.

or

JUMP START RECIPE OPTION: Thai Chicken Wrap (page 193)

SNACK
¼ avocado with Himalayan salt or unrefined sea salt
1 large tomato, sliced

6 gluten-free seeded crackers

or

JUMP START RECIPE OPTION: Lime Guacamole (page 157) and Crispy Crackers (page 126)

DINNER

Salmon and Sweet Potato
1 tablespoon coconut oil
1 cup mixed vegetables
Himalayan salt or unrefined salt and freshly ground black pepper
6 ounces grilled salmon (or swap in another fish or grilled chicken)
½ cooked sweet potato

INSTRUCTIONS: Heat the oil in a skillet over medium heat. Add the vegetables and sauté until softened but still al dente; season with salt and pepper. Add to plate with the grilled salmon and sweet potato.

or

JUMP START RECIPE OPTION: Grilled Salmon Kebabs (page 205) with Sweet Potato Bowl (page 161)

DAY 5

BREAKFAST
1 cup strawberries
2 eggs, cooked to your liking
1 piece cooked nitrate-free turkey bacon

or

JUMP START RECIPE OPTION: Cacao Pancakes (page 109)

SNACK
Raw sugar snap peas
1 tablespoon hummus

LUNCH
Mango Shrimp
    1 teaspoon olive oil
    6 ounces shrimp (or swap in scallops, white
        fish, or chicken)
    Himalayan salt or unrefined salt and freshly
        ground black pepper
    1 cup mixed lettuce
    1 mango, sliced (or another fruit of choice)
    Juice of ½ lime
    1 tablespoon feta cheese or ¼ avocado

INSTRUCTIONS: Heat the oil in a skillet over medium heat. Add the shrimp and cook until opaque throughout. Season with salt and pepper. Arrange the lettuce and mango on a plate and top with the shrimp. Finish with the lime juice and feta or avocado.

or

JUMP START RECIPE OPTION: Shrimp with Mango Salsa (page 215)

SNACK
    6 macadamia nuts
    Small piece of fruit (such as an apple,
        orange, peach, pear, or ½ banana)

or

JUMP START RECIPE OPTION: Peaches 'n' Cream (page 135)

DINNER
Halibut with Snap Peas
    1 tablespoon coconut oil
    1 cup sugar snap peas
    1 tablespoon sliced, oil-packed sun-dried
        tomatoes
    Himalayan salt or unrefined salt and freshly
        ground black pepper
    6 ounces halibut (or swap in another white
        fish or chicken)
    Juice of ½ lemon

INSTRUCTIONS: Heat the oil in a skillet over medium heat. Add the sugar snap peas and sun-dried tomatoes and sauté until the peas are crisp-tender. Season with salt and pepper. Season the halibut with salt and pepper, add to the pan, and cook on both sides until cooked through. Place on a plate and finish with the lemon juice.

or

JUMP START RECIPE OPTION: Lemon Halibut with Caper Sauce (page 207) with Grilled Asparagus (page 163)

DAY 6

BREAKFAST
Portobello Scramble
    1 teaspoon olive oil
    1 portobello mushroom, stem removed
        and chopped
    2 eggs, beaten
    Himalayan salt or unrefined salt and freshly
        ground black pepper
    1 tablespoon goat cheese

INSTRUCTIONS: Heat the oil in a skillet over medium heat. Add the mushroom and cook until softened. Add the eggs and scramble to your liking. Season with salt and pepper and top with the goat cheese.

or

JUMP START RECIPE OPTION: Portobello Poached Eggs (page 121)

SNACK

½ cucumber, diced
Handful cherry tomatoes, halved
1 tablespoon diced red onion (optional)
1 tablespoon feta cheese
1 tablespoon red wine vinegar

INSTRUCTIONS: Toss all the ingredients in a bowl.

or

JUMP START RECIPE OPTION: 1 cup Butternut Squash Soup (page 148) topped with 1 tablespoon goat cheese

LUNCH

1 cup lettuce
1 cup chopped bell pepper
1 tablespoon chopped cilantro
6 ounces cooked shrimp (or swap in scallops, white fish, or chicken)
¼ avocado, sliced
Juice of ½ lime
Juice of ½ lemon
Himalayan salt or unrefined salt and freshly ground black pepper

INSTRUCTIONS: Place the lettuce on a plate. Top with the pepper, cilantro, shrimp, and avocado. Squeeze the lemon and lime juice on top and season with salt and pepper.

or

JUMP START RECIPE OPTION: Shrimp Ceviche (page 213)

SNACK

1 tablespoon no-sugar-added almond butter
1 small pear or other fruit

DINNER

Chicken with Mushrooms and Tomatoes

1 tablespoon coconut oil
½ onion, sliced
1 cup sliced mushrooms (your choice)
½ cup cherry tomatoes, sliced
6 ounces chicken (or swap in lean red meat, pork, turkey, or fish)
Himalayan salt or unrefined salt and freshly ground black pepper
Juice of ½ lemon

INSTRUCTIONS: Heat the oil in a skillet over medium heat. Add the onion and sauté until translucent. Add the mushrooms and cherry tomatoes and sauté until mushrooms are softened. Season the chicken with salt and pepper and cook until cooked through. Serve with the lemon juice squeezed on top.

or

JUMP START RECIPE OPTION: Chicken and Rice with a Bite (page 183)

DAY 7

BREAKFAST

Cinnamon Apple Oats
  ½ cup cooked oatmeal
  ¼ apple, diced
  1 tablespoon coconut oil
  Sprinkle of cinnamon
  2 slices cooked, nitrate-free turkey bacon

INSTRUCTIONS: Mix the oatmeal with the apple and oil. Top with a sprinkle of cinnamon and serve with the turkey bacon.

  or

JUMP START RECIPE OPTION: Applesauce Overnight Oats (page 102) with 1 slice nitrate-free turkey bacon

SNACK

Balsamic Turkey and Melon
  ½ cup cubed melon
  4 ounces sliced smoked turkey breast
  1 tablespoon walnuts
  1 tablespoon balsamic vinegar

INSTRUCTIONS: Toss all the ingredients in a bowl and serve.

LUNCH

Turkey Salad
  6 ounces cooked, sliced turkey breast (or swap in grilled chicken)
  1 cup shredded romaine lettuce

  1 slice cooked, nitrate-free turkey bacon, crumbled
  1 tomato, diced
  Juice of ½ lemon
  Himalayan salt or unrefined salt and freshly ground black pepper to taste

INSTRUCTIONS: Toss all the ingredients in a bowl and serve.

  or

JUMP START RECIPE OPTION: Turkey Bacon Club Wrap (page 106)

SNACK

Spinach and Hard-Boiled Egg
  1 tablespoon sliced almonds
  1 tablespoon feta cheese
  ½ cup spinach
  1 hard-boiled egg, sliced
  Juice of ½ lemon

INSTRUCTIONS: Toss all the ingredients in a bowl and serve.

  or

JUMP START RECIPE OPTION: Spinach Stuffed Mushrooms (page 173)

DINNER

Spinach Chicken
  1 tablespoon extra-virgin olive oil
  1 to 2 garlic cloves, diced
  ½ onion, sliced

1 celery stalk, chopped
1 carrot, sliced
6 ounces chicken (or swap in grilled fish, pork, or lean red meat)
1 cup spinach
Juice of ½ lemon

or

JUMP START RECIPE OPTION: Chicken and Kale Soup (page 154) with 1 tablespoon Lime Guacamole (page 157)

INSTRUCTIONS: Heat the oil in a skillet over medium heat. Add the garlic and onion and sauté until translucent. Add the celery and carrots and sauté until slightly softened. Add the chicken and cook until cooked through. Add the spinach, cover and cook until wilted. Transfer to a plate and top with the lemon juice.

*If hungry before bed, add a small protein/fat course (no carbs) such as:

3 ounces salmon
6 macadamia nuts
½ cup cottage cheese
2 eggs

IT'S BETTER TO BUILD A MEAL THAN TO SKIP A MEAL

Sometimes meetings go longer than expected, traffic stands still, and reservations get pushed back for friends who are running late. That is why I always keep healthful options stashed in my bag, car, or purse depending on where I am going. If you are at work, keep a little stash at your desk. On-hand go-to snacks are a must to help you avoid the office candy machine or fast-food runs. Good things to keep handy include almonds, healthy protein bars, apples, protein powder, tuna packets, and a lot of water.

When your only reasonable choice is a convenience store, you still can build a meal that contains protein, carbs, and healthful fat that won't sabotage your waistline. I am not suggesting making convenience stores or fast-food chains part of your daily meals. But when you find yourself in this sort of bind, you'll find you have options in some of the most surprising places. It is always better to *build* a meal than skip a meal.

Protein options:

Hard-boiled eggs
Cottage cheese
Turkey jerky
Plain Greek yogurt
Protein bars (check sugar and calorie content—eat just half if they are high)
Protein shakes
Turkey sandwich (toss the bread)

Carbohydrate options:

Fresh fruit and veggie sticks
Fresh fruit salad from a deli section

Fat options:

Unsalted and unsweetened nuts
Nut butters
Avocado
Seeds

7 TIPS FOR TACKLING CRAVINGS

EVEN I sometimes crave sugar or carbs. I don't avoid them completely; I just make sure not to overdo it. (Remember the majority rules: once you are at your goal and have made it a lifestyle, it is easier to maintain, so keep it clean about 80 percent of the time, and it is OK to have a treat every now and then.) Here are some of my favorite strategies for tackling cravings:

1. Drink a glass of water. Then wait a few minutes and see if the craving goes away. If not, try one of the following tips.
2. Have a little healthy fat, and if you can, some protein. Six to eight almonds usually does the trick, but if you really need something more, a little piece of fish or chicken with the almonds will go a long way to putting those cravings to bed.
3. Add a little Himalayan pink salt or unrefined sea salt to your food. It contains no calories and will give you a flavor boost. You'll be surprised how the salt can satisfy your craving without sacrificing your healthy diet! I know sodium gets a bad rap, but it's actually an important part of an unprocessed diet (see page 65 to see why).
4. Take a walk or read a magazine. Get your mind and body occupied—away from temptation.
5. Do the Posture Squeeze, one of my favorite ways of improving posture and alleviating back pain. See page 272 to learn how.
6. Try an unprocessed treat such as a baked apple sprinkled with cinnamon or one of my dessert recipes (see pages 223 to 236).
7. Get outside and spend a few minutes in nature. Enjoy the fresh air and the warmth of the sun hitting your skin. A few minutes of sun is the best way to produce vitamin D, and it rejuvenates the body as well.

TRAVELING OR EATING OUT? SWAP IT OUT!

With a little forethought, you can sail through any challenge. When I make plans to eat out, I try to research the restaurant a little beforehand. Many list their menus online. If not, call the restaurant and ask about their offerings. For the most part, it isn't that hard getting something healthy. Most places can prepare a lean protein (such as chicken or fish) and some sort of vegetable for you even if it isn't listed on the menu that way. Create your own restaurant meal by choosing a dish that contains the proper balance of protein, fat, and healthful carbohydrates.

Order a serving of protein, choose a salad (or vegetable side) with an olive oil-based dressing on the side, and you are pretty much good to go. There you have your protein, healthy fats, and healthy (non-starchy) carbs.

When traveling, you have so many choices for on-the-go snacks: protein bars and shakes, nuts, seeds, nut butters, fresh fruit, tuna packets, and raw veggies. If you need to rely on a chain or fast-food restaurant, order eggs, yogurt sans granola, chicken, or even grilled shrimp fajitas. Plain baked potatoes are OK in a pinch; upgrade to a sweet potato when available; and avoid the french fries, as tempting as they may be.

STILL HUNGRY?

WHEN you are eating healthfully, you need enough food so your body can maintain and repair itself and promote the growth of lean muscle mass, while at the same time minimizing fat storage. Part of any initial hunger you might experience on the program may have to do with getting used to this new way of eating. If you are used to 1,000-plus-calorie fast-food meals for lunch, it is going to take a few days for your body to adjust.

My first line of attack: Try upping your veggies. Raw or steamed vegetables are unlimited and encouraged. Eat away! Plus, I will give you so many great recipes to make vegetables your new food of choice. If that does not completely work, add some more fat—5 to 8 almonds is a good start, or increase the protein portion of your meal. Do not add more starchy carbohydrates or sugars, as they will only make you hungrier. Fats and protein will do the most to help curb further cravings, and remember to drink lots of water. Lots of times, hunger is thirst in disguise.

Taking some rest is another option. When you're overtired, your system goes out of whack, and that includes your metabolism. If you've got the opportunity for a midday nap, take it. Otherwise make a commitment to try to get some extra shut-eye over the next couple of days. Studies have found that individuals who sleep a consistent seven to nine hours a night experience fewer weight problems.

"While I'm not advocating making fast food a regular part of your nutrition plan, there are ways to make smart choices and get 'food fast.'"

Burger or Chicken Chain

- Small hamburger or grilled chicken sandwich
- No cheese, no "special" sauces, and get rid of the bun (ask if they'll make you a "bun" out of lettuce leaves)
- Avoid mayonnaise-based side orders such as coleslaw and potato salad
- Avoid anything breaded or fried

Mexican Chain

- Choose grilled chicken or shrimp and any vegetables you can find, with a small amount of avocado
- Leave off the cheese, sour cream, and beans
- If a taco is the only option, get rid of the wrapper and eat just the filling
- Stay away from hard-shelled options like tacos or tostadas
- Don't even think about getting a margarita

Sandwich Chain

- Choose lean meats (turkey, chicken, roast beef) and toss the bread
- Stick with mustard or a little oil and vinegar as your condiments

- Avoid cheeses, sauces, and mayonnaise that love to get slathered on
- Add as many vegetables as possible

Asian Chain

- Stick to steamed, roasted, or broiled entrees
- Ask if they have brown rice (not fried rice)
- Order sashimi (raw fish without the rice)
- Ask for stir-fries with little or no oil

Italian Chain

- Order fish; broiled or baked is best
- Find out if there is a gluten-free whole-grain pasta option
- Avoid cream sauces and breaded options like eggplant Parmesan
- Get a big salad with Italian dressing on the side
- Add extra veggies to whatever you get

Smoothie Chain

- Choose the smallest serving and check the calorie chart
- Stick to lighter options that use water and mostly frozen fruits rather than fruit juices
- Add protein boosts where available (ask to see the ingredients of their protein powder)
- Stay away from soy milk and peanut butter
- Definitely pass on smoothies using ice cream or sherbet

BEING VEGETARIAN ON THE 7 DAY JUMP START

WITH the flood of documentaries and celebrities promoting plant-based diets for better health, *vegetarian* and *vegan* seem to be buzz words lately. There are some compelling arguments for a plant-based diet—including the possible prevention of type 2 diabetes, heart disease, and cancer—but before you dive in headfirst, do your research and know what you are getting into so you can make the best decision for yourself.

People are constantly asking me if I can swap out the animal proteins for vegetarian proteins in my nutrition plan. I'll be frank with you: following a vegetarian diet will take a solid commitment with a bit of extra thinking and planning. Going out to eat at a restaurant or a friend's house for dinner will require more preparation. You must be willing to eat ahead of time, share your food preferences with friends, and be prepared to ask restaurants to adjust meals for you.

The easiest way to be a vegetarian on my 7 Day Jump Start is as an **ovo-lacto vegetarian**, meaning you include both eggs and dairy in your diet. Being an **ovo vegetarian** (including eggs but no dairy) or **lacto vegetarian** (including dairy but no eggs) is more of a challenge. **Vegans**, who follow a plant-based diet with no eggs or dairy (and some vegans omit honey as well) face the biggest challenge in getting good-quality protein without maxing out in the carb department. Although I respect the vegan diet, because it is so hard to get lean eating this way, my nutrition program does not include a vegan option. But if veganism is a personal commitment for you, do supplement with a quality plant-based protein powder. And keep in mind that whether you're a meat-eater or vegetarian, your protein needs will increase when you start a fitness routine, as resistance training and endurance workouts can rapidly break down muscle protein.

It's a fact that many vegetarian protein options and even more vegan options are lower-quality proteins and heavy in carbohydrates, which can lead to weight gain if not balanced with the proper amount of fats and high-quality protein. Many vegetarians and vegans are perfect examples of people who are eating a lot of healthy foods, but not eating healthy as far as fat loss is concerned. Very few body types respond well to a very carb-heavy diet.

Here's the problem: there are almost no plant-based sources of pure protein. For example, you can eat a piece of chicken or fish or 3 to 4 egg whites and easily get 24 to 30 grams of protein, 0 to 1 gram of fat, and 1 to 2 grams of carbs in about 120 to 130 calories. Not true of vegetarian proteins. Even quinoa, which vegetarians and vegans love as a complete protein, has four times as many carbs as protein. So to get 25 grams of protein from quinoa, you'd end up eating 109 grams of carbs and more than 600 calories in total. It's hard to lose weight and get lean when you have to eat 600 calories to get the same 25 grams of protein those 120 to 130 calories of animal protein provide.

Even vegetables like spinach that have a lot of protein as a percentage of weight have no density. What I mean by density is that you would have to eat more than 25 cups of spinach to get 25 grams of protein! Beans are another vegetarian protein source that has a lot of carbs, and I don't have to tell you that most people can't handle eating a lot of beans on a daily basis. I see a lot of

continues

continued

vegetarians and vegans lean heavily on soy, which has its own set of issues as a primary protein source (see page 81).

Protein aside, vegetarians and especially vegans, might consider supplementing with vitamin B12, as the only natural sources of this vitamin are from meat, dairy, and eggs. If you're not eating dairy, make sure you get good-quality calcium from sources such as coconut milk, chickpeas, broccoli and leafy greens, and figs. Your body has to have vitamin D to absorb the calcium it needs, so if you're not getting sun on a regular basis, you might want to supplement. Zinc is a biggie for metabolism, immunity, and overall good health. Vegetarians can need up to 50 percent more zinc than meat eaters because the zinc found in plants isn't absorbed by the body as well as animal sources. Plant-based sources include whole grains (make sure they are gluten-free, which means no wheat, barley, or rye), miso, legumes, nuts, seeds, and egg and dairy products.

I eat a plant-*based* diet, but I do eat fish, shrimp, eggs, and on occasion, chicken and turkey, and I supplement with protein powder with my workouts, as quality lean protein is important to stay satisfied, lean, and healthy. I want to support you in losing weight and staying healthy with whatever lifestyle decisions you make. For that reason, I've included vegetarian swaps for all seven days of the jump start. But do keep in mind that vegetarians who do eat eggs and dairy often fare better than others when it comes to weight loss in all my plans. Eggs, dairy, and protein powder are an important part of a successful vegetarian 7 Day Jump Start, and those who go the **pescatarian** route (adding fish to their diet) fare the best. I know this is a very passionate subject for many people. In the end, if it works for you, keep doing it!

What Won't Work

- Only restricting calories (but still not eating the right foods)
- Counting calories too much
- Only eating one or two big meals a day
- Maintaining the same unhealthy eating habits while trying to cardio away the calories
- Eating a lot of overly processed "diet" foods (shakes, bars, frozen meals)
- Eating fat-free foods and sugar-free processed foods
- Eliminating an entire macronutrient (such as no-fat or no-carb plans)
- Taking diet supplements (they tend to be high in caffeine and dehydrating)
- Eating on autopilot
- Trying to exercise your way out of poor nutrition habits

What *Will* Work

- Eliminating processed foods
- Eating naturally unprocessed foods
- Limiting processed and other "empty" carbohydrates
- Changing the types of carbohydrates you *do* eat
- Eating smaller quantities 5 to 6 times a day
- Favoring organic foods
- Eliminating or reducing corn- and soy-based products

PART 2

THE
RECIPES

NOW it's time to get into the kitchen, cook up some amazing unprocessed food, and have some fun! You'll be starting out with the recipes I've chosen for the meal plan (page 83); those remaining will become a part of your everyday menus beyond the seven days as you turn this way of eating into a lifestyle.

My recipes are all based on the natural ingredients and principles of the Jump Start I've shared with you in the first section of the book. They're simple to make and really, really tasty. No deprivation just because you've chosen to eat healthy! All are gluten-free, with none of those quick-fix fake substitutes that doom many diets to failure.

From twists on old favorite like chocolate mousse made with avocado to reinvented classics such as crustless quiche and waffles that skip the wheat, there's something to please every eater. All are quick, with some that you can put together in five minutes—even the busiest of us have five minutes for a nourishing meal!

The whole family will love what you're making, and they'll happily join you in unprocessing your diet because they won't even know what they're eating is healthy! The hardest part will be choosing which ones to make and sticking to one serving. But unlike many "diet" recipes, these contain real, unprocessed fat, which goes a long way to keeping your portions under control. Plus, they are full of vegetables, which makes them nutrient-dense and really hydrating. I don't skimp on the salt, but I make sure to use nutrient-rich Himalayan salt or unrefined sea salt, as it brings out the flavor without the added calories. Your food has to have flavor for you to love it! In place of table sugar, I've swapped in delicious, unprocessed sweeteners including maple syrup, agave nectar, and coconut sugar. When you go unprocessed, you'll find a little dessert goes a long way without the urge for seconds and thirds.

Now you can literally "eat your excuses" and move on!

8
BREAKFAST

APPLESAUCE OVERNIGHT OATS

YIELD: 2 servings

Skipping breakfast is not an option on my Jump Start. But *making* breakfast in the morning is optional. For days when there just isn't time, invest a couple of minutes on your morning meal the night before and your rewards will be sweet. These applesauce oats can be served either cold or warmed.

Ingredients:

- ½ cup rolled oats
- ½ cup unsweetened almond milk
- ½ cup unsweetened applesauce (store-bought or homemade; applesauce recipe on page 103)
- ½ teaspoon cinnamon or apple pie spice (optional, depending on applesauce)
- Pinch of sea salt

Directions:

➤ Stir all ingredients together in a medium bowl. Divide mixture between two sealable containers (such as mason jars).

➤ Place in the fridge overnight (or for several hours). In the morning, eat cold or warm up for 1-2 minutes in the microwave.

TIP: If you don't have time to make your own applesauce, look for a no-sugar-added brand, an organic one if possible.

SERVES 2

Calories: 157/Calories from fat: 20
Fat: 2.2g, Protein: 4.1 g, Total Carb: 30g, Fiber: 5.4g, Sugars: 12g, Sodium: 95mg, Vitamin A: 185mg, Vitamin C: 1mg, Calcium: 75mg, Iron: 1.2mg

NATURALLY SWEET APPLESAUCE

YIELD: 2¼ cups

Making your own gives you the freshest tasting applesauce, and you get to flavor it just as you like—cinnamon alone, or accented with nutmeg and allspice too. As you unprocess your diet, you'll come to appreciate the natural sweet and tart flavor of apples—no need to add sugar to your apples to turn them into applesauce!

Ingredients:

- 6 apples, golden delicious preferred
- 1 cup water
- 1 tablespoon fresh lemon juice
- ¼ teaspoon cinnamon
- ¼ teaspoon nutmeg, optional
- ¼ teaspoon allspice, optional

Directions:

➤ Peel and core apples and cut into quarters. Place them in a saucepan with the water and lemon juice, then bring to a boil over high heat, about 1 minute. Reduce to a simmer and cook, stirring occasionally until broken down and thickened, about 45 minutes.

➤ Take off the heat and stir in the cinnamon and other spices if using. Let cool to room temperature, then refrigerate until ready to use.

➤ Store in an airtight container in the refrigerator for up to 5 days.

PER ¼ CUP SERVING:
Calories: 65/Calories from fat: 2
Fat: 0.2g, Protein: 0.3g, Total carb: 15.6g, Fiber: 2.8g, Sugars: 11.4, Sodium: 2mg, Vitamin A: 58mg, Vitamin C: 1mg, Calcium: 8mg, Iron: 0.2mg

SLOW COOKER COCONUTTY PEAR OATMEAL

SERVES 4 (serving size: ¾ cup)

This rich-tasting, slightly sweet breakfast is the perfect way to start your day. And the best thing about it is all the work is done the night before! Just add your ingredients to a slow cooker before you jump under the covers, set the timer for eight to nine hours, and wake up to the warming aromas of cinnamon oats.

Ingredients:

- 2 tablespoons organic grass-fed butter
- 2 medium ripe pears, halved, pitted, and sliced into ¼" wedges
- 1-2 teaspoons ground cinnamon
- 1 cup rolled oats
- 1 cup coconut flakes, unsweetened
- Pinch of salt
- 3 cups water

Directions:

➤ Break up butter into smaller pieces and lay on bottom of crockpot. Slice pears and lay on top of the butter, and sprinkle cinnamon on top of pears. Pour in oatmeal, coconut, salt, and then the water. Do not stir.

➤ Turn crockpot on low and cook overnight for 8-9 hours until rich and smooth.

Calories: 285/Calories from fat: 152
Fat: 16.9g, Protein: 4.9g, Total carb: 30.8g, Fiber: 7g, Sugars: 10g, Sodium: 30mg, Vitamin A: 176mg, Vitamin C: 4mg, Calcium: 24mg, Iron: 1.1mg

RASPBERRY TWIST SMOOTHIE

DAY
4
BREAKFAST

SERVES 1

Creamy, frothy, and lightly sweet, this pretty in pink smoothie is a snap to put together and goes a long way to keeping you satisfied through the morning.

Ingredients:

½ cup frozen raspberries
½ banana, sliced, frozen
Juice of 1 small orange
¼ cup unsweetened almond milk
¼ cup 2% Greek yogurt
1 tablespoon almond butter

Directions:

➤ Place all ingredients into blender and blend on high until smooth.

TIP: Look for overripe bananas on sale at the supermarket; peel and store the bananas in the freezer in ziplock bags. That way you'll be set for smoothie-making any time you like!

Calories: 247/Calories from fat: 92
Fat: 10.1g, Protein: 10g, Total carb: 32.5g, Fiber: 6.3g, Sugars: 18g, Sodium: 65mg, Vitamin A: 312mg, Vitamin C: 45mg, Calcium: 145mg, Iron: 1.4mg

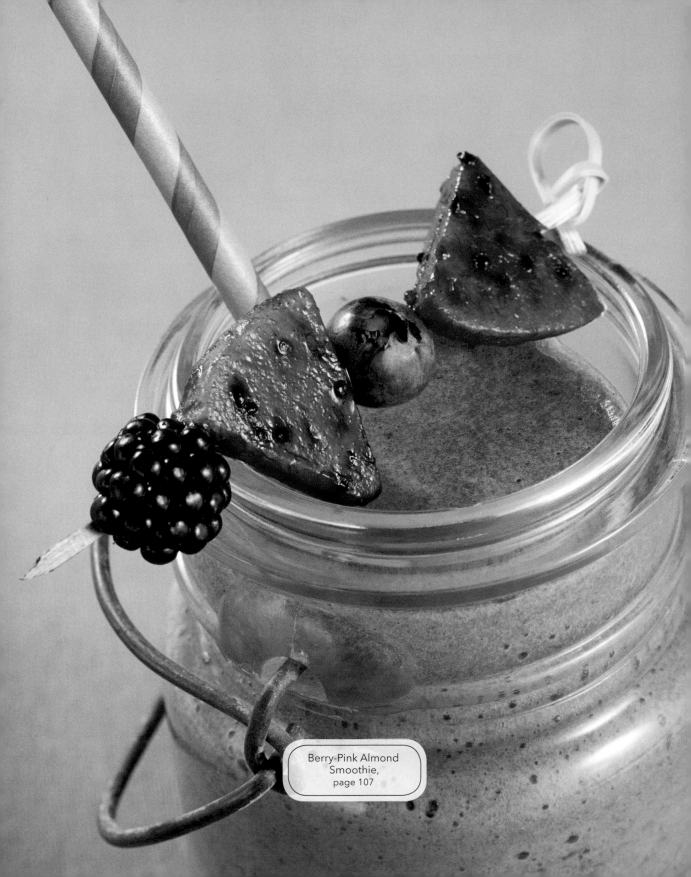

Berry-Pink Almond
Smoothie,
page 107

BERRY-PINK ALMOND SMOOTHIE

SERVES 1

This fruity smoothie uses the amazing pitaya, or dragon fruit, hailed as a superfood for its antioxidant content. This exotic cactus fruit, brilliant pink and shaped like a rosebud with dragon-like spikes, is mildly sweet and crunchy. To get to the fruit, slice it in half lengthwise and scoop out the flesh. The white part with the seeds is what you want to eat. Look for dragon fruit in the freezer section of your local grocer or natural foods store.

Ingredients:

- ½ cup frozen mixed berries (strawberry, raspberry, blueberry, blackberry)
- 3.5 ounces Pitaya/Dragon Fruit (found in the frozen section of most natural food stores), peeled and cut into ½-inch chunks
- Juice from 1 orange
- 1 tablespoon almond butter
- 1 cup ice
- 1 teaspoon pure almond extract

Directions:

- ➤ Place all ingredients into blender and blend on high until smooth.

Calories: 227/Calories from fat: 77
Fat: 8.5g, Protein: 5.7g, Total carb: 32.8g, Fiber: 5.6g, Sugars: 10.9g, Sodium: 1mg, Vitamin A: 137mg, Vitamin C: 125mg, Calcium: 47mg, Iron: 1.1mg

ANTIOXIDANT SMOOTHIE

SERVES 2

Not too sweet, very refreshing, and packed with all of the green goodness spinach offers. You'll love this smoothie either for breakfast or as an afternoon snack.

Ingredients:

½ cup pumpkin seeds
1 cup frozen mixed berries
½ cup unsweetened
    pomegranate juice
½ cup unsweetened almond milk
1 cup spinach
½ tablespoon hulled hemp seeds

Directions:

➤ Place pumpkin seeds in the blender and blend on high until they become like a powder. Place all the remaining ingredients in blender and mix until smooth.

Calories: 267/Calories from fat: 148
Fat: 16.5g, Protein: 11g, Total carb: 23.8g, Fiber: 5.2g, Sugars: 14g, Sodium: 78mg, Vitamin A: 586mg, Vitamin C: 13mg, Calcium: 96mg, Iron: 3.6mg

GRAIN-FREE CACAO PANCAKES

SERVES 5 (serving size: 2 pancakes)

Who says you need wheat to make a pancake? In fact, you don't need flour at all! Banana pancakes are becoming big with unprocessed food eaters, and for good reason—they're high in protein and just a little sweet, with a little coconut oil providing the perfect balance of fat.

Ingredients:

- 1 large ripe banana, peeled and sliced
- 4 large eggs
- 2 tablespoons coconut oil, melted
- 3 tablespoons raw cacao powder

Directions:

➤ Place the banana, eggs, cacao powder, and melted coconut oil in a food processor or blender. Blend until smooth.

➤ Heat skillet or griddle on medium-low heat. Brush with coconut oil to prevent sticking.

➤ Pour batter onto skillet, about 3 tablespoons for each pancake. Cook until the top bubbles, and the bottom is golden, approximately 5 minutes. Flip, and cook another 2 minutes.

TIP: Make sure to buy unsweetened cacao powder, not the one used for hot chocolate, as that's filled with sugar.

Calories: 167/Calories from fat: 97
Fat: 11.1g, Protein: 7.2g, Total carb: 10.9g, Fiber: 3.1g, Sugars: 3.3g, Sodium: 60mg, Vitamin A: 257mg, Vitamin C: 2mg, Calcium: 17mg, Iron: 0.7mg

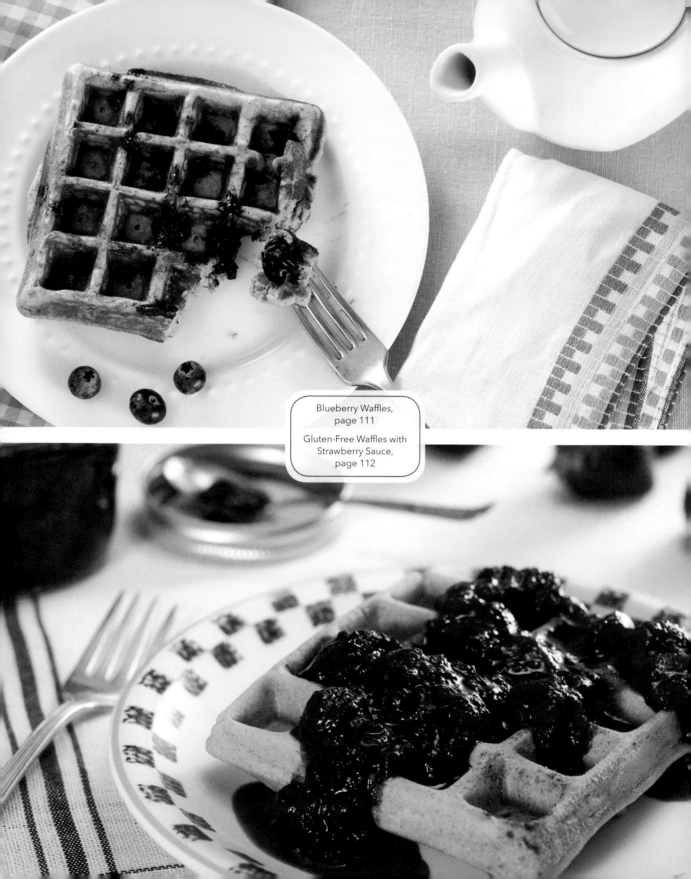

Blueberry Waffles,
page 111

Gluten-Free Waffles with
Strawberry Sauce,
page 112

BLUEBERRY WAFFLES

MAKES 4 6" round waffles or **5 4"** square waffles

Who needs syrup when you have waffles that taste this good? Blueberries and bananas make these waffles moist, and almond butter adds protein and a hint of almond flavor. For even more almond flavor, add a couple of drops of almond extract.

Ingredients:

- 3 large eggs
- 2 ripe bananas
- 3 tablespoons almond butter, plain, without salt added
- ½ teaspoon pure vanilla extract
- ½ teaspoon pumpkin pie spice
- ¼ cup almond flour
- ½ cup tapioca flour
- ½ cup, fresh blueberries
- 2 tablespoons coconut oil for cooking

Directions:

➤ Preheat the waffle iron according to the manufacturer's instructions.

➤ Combine the eggs, bananas, almond butter, vanilla extract, pumpkin pie spice, almond flour, and tapioca flour in a blender and blend until smooth.

➤ Transfer the batter to a medium bowl and fold in the blueberries.

➤ Once the waffle iron is hot, brush coconut oil on the top and bottom of the iron. Pour a heaping ½ cup batter to each waffle (if making a 4-inch square) or a heaping ⅔ cup amount (if making a 6-inch round). Repeat process with coconut oil and batter until all the batter is used. Serve immediately or cool to room temperature and freeze in an airtight container for up to 1 month.

PER 1 6-INCH WAFFLE:

Calories: 342/Calories from fat: 181

Fat: 20.4g, Protein: 9.7g, Total carb: 35.5g, Fiber: 4.3g, Sugars: 10.3g, Sodium: 50mg, Vitamin A: 273mg, Vitamin C: 63mg, Calcium: 63mg, Iron: 1.5mg

GLUTEN-FREE WAFFLES WITH STRAWBERRY SAUCE

SERVES 6

How can a gluten-free waffle taste so good? Hearty oat flour gives it stick-to-your-ribs substance, and only the most wholesome of ingredients makes for a waffle that you can turn to again and again. A maple syrup–sweetened strawberry sauce jazzes up your waffles, leaving you wondering how you ever ate the fake stuff!

Ingredients:

1½ cup gluten fr ee oat flour
2 teaspoon baking powder
¼ teaspoon Himalayan salt
Pinch ground cinnamon
¾ cup unsweetened almond milk
¼ cup + 1 tablespoon melted
    coconut oil
2 large eggs
2 tablespoons grade B organic
    maple syrup
1 teaspoon pure vanilla extract

Strawberry Sauce, for serving
    (recipe page 113)

Directions:

➤ In a large bowl, whisk together the oat flour, baking powder, salt, and cinnamon until combined.

➤ In a separate bowl, whisk together the almond milk, coconut oil, eggs, maple syrup, and vanilla.

➤ Pour wet ingredients into dry and stir until just combined (still a little lumpy). Let batter sit for 10 minutes.

➤ Heat waffle iron.

➤ After the 10 minutes, stir batter one more time just to move it around a little.

➤ Pour batter into center of waffle iron and let it spread to the edges.

➤ Cook until golden. Depending upon machine, cooking time will vary. My waffles took 4 minutes to cook until golden brown. Remove when done and let cool slightly. Do not stack waffles or they will lose their crispness.

Calories: 275/Calories from fat: 135
Fat: 15.6g, Protein: 6.2g, Total carb: 27.7g, Fiber: 3.6g, Sugars: 5g, Sodium: 293mg, Vitamin A: 163mg, Vitamin C: 0mg,
Calcium: 85mg, Iron: 1.6mg

STRAWBERRY SAUCE

YIELDS: 2½ cups

You can use grade B organic maple syrup in this recipe instead of the coconut nectar.

Ingredients:

- 3 cups fresh strawberries washed and hulled
- 3 tablespoon coconut nectar
- 1 teaspoon pure vanilla extract
- Zest of 2 lemons

Directions:

➤ Place strawberries in a medium pot and smash with meat tenderizer or potato masher (or anything that will fit in the pot and has a flat bottom).

➤ Add coconut nectar or grade B organic maple syrup, vanilla, and zest and cook over medium heat for about 12-15 minutes. The mixture will thicken slightly.

➤ Spoon desired amount over waffles upon serving.

➤ Store sauce in refrigerator for up to 5 days, or freeze your leftovers.

PER ¼ CUP:

Calories: 19/Calories from fat: 0.9

Fat: 0.1g, Protein: 0.3g, Total carb: 3.9g, Fiber: 0.7g, Sugars: 2.9g, Sodium: 1mg, Vitamin A: 0mg, Vitamin C: 29mg, Calcium: 7mg, Iron: 0.1mg

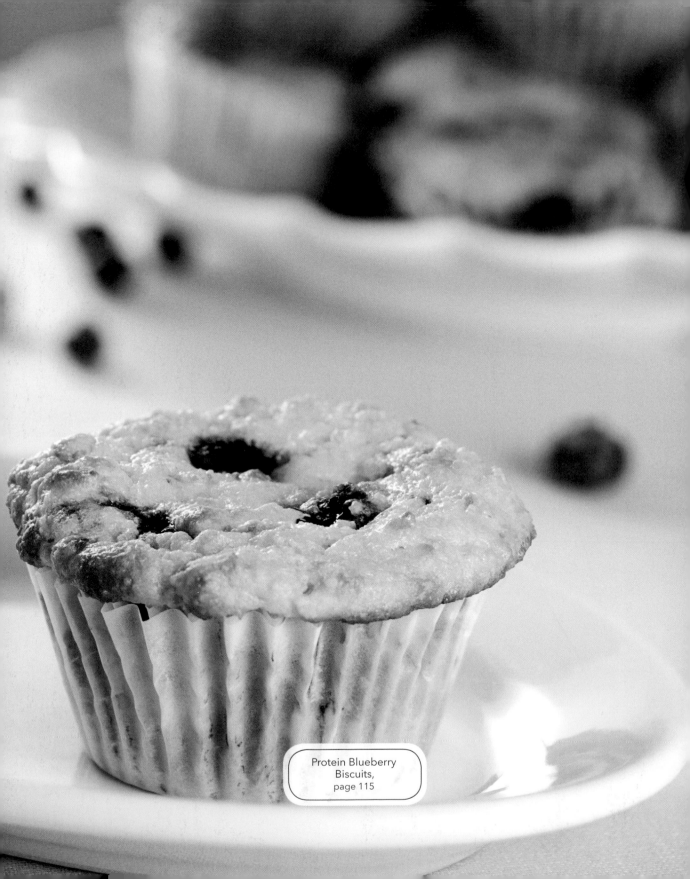

Protein Blueberry
Biscuits,
page 115

PROTEIN BLUEBERRY BISCUITS

SERVES 12 (serving size: 1 biscuit)

These biscuits pack in the protein, and applesauce and blueberries are all that's needed to give them a hint of natural sweetness.

Ingredients:

2 cups almond flour
1 cup oats—quick or regular oats, plain
⅔ cup unsweetened applesauce (see page 103)
1 teaspoon baking powder
1 teaspoon baking soda
½ teaspoon Himalayan salt
1½ cups 2% plain Greek yogurt
2 large eggs, lightly beaten
2 tablespoons organic, unsalted, grass-fed butter, melted and slightly cooled
1 teaspoon pure vanilla extract
1 cup fresh blueberries

Directions:

➤ Heat oven to 350°. Line a standard-sized non-stick muffin tin with paper liners.
➤ Combine flour, oats, baking powder, baking soda, and salt in a large bowl.
➤ Combine applesauce, yogurt, eggs, butter, and vanilla in a second bowl. Fold yogurt mixture into dry mixture; stir to combine completely. Gently fold in blueberries.
➤ Spoon, or use an ice cream scoop or pour into muffin tins filling until ¾ full. Bake until top is golden and a toothpick inserted into the center of a biscuit comes out clean, about 30 to 35 minutes. Let cool in pan about 10 minutes before transferring biscuits to a cooling rack to cool completely.

TIP: Freeze some of your biscuits right after they've cooled. Take one out when you get up in the morning, then pop it into the toaster oven to reheat.

Calories: 220/Calories from fat: 124
Fat: 13.7g, Protein: 9.4g, Total carb: 14.9g, Fiber: 3.7g, Sugars: 6g, Sodium: 235mg, Vitamin A: 132mg, Vitamin C: 1mg, Calcium: 89mg, Iron: 1.2mg, Sugars: 5g, Sodium: 101mg, Vitamin A: 357mg, Vitamin C: 3mg, Calcium: 14mg, Iron: 0.5mg

BLUEBERRY LEMON MUFFINS

YIELDS: 12 muffins

Yes, you can still have muffins! These super-moist, high-protein muffins are so scrumptious, you won't even think to miss the high-calorie varieties. A little lemon makes the berry flavor really pop!

Ingredients:

- 6 large eggs
- ½ cup unsalted, grass-fed butter or coconut oil, melted
- 1 teaspoon pure vanilla extract
- 3 tablespoons grade B maple syrup
- 1 lemon, juice and zest
- ½ cup coconut flour
- ¼ teaspoon sea salt
- ¼ teaspoon baking soda
- 1 cup fresh blueberries

Directions:

➤ Preheat oven to 350 degrees. Line a standard-sized non-stick muffin tin with paper liners.

➤ Whisk the eggs, butter or coconut oil, pure vanilla, maple syrup, lemon juice and zest together in a large bowl. Sift in the coconut flour, sea salt, and baking soda, and whisk until well combined. Batter will look lumpy at first but keep whisking until smooth and thickened. Gently fold in the blueberries.

➤ Fill the lined muffin tin cups ¾ full with mix and bake 35–40 minutes. Let cool slightly in pan, about 10 minutes before transferring to a wire rack to cool completely.

*Nutrition calculated with coconut oil
Calories: 157/Calories from fat: 107
Fat: 12.3g, Protein: 3.8g, Total carb: 8.6g, Fiber: 2g, Sugars: 5g, Sodium: 101mg, Vitamin A: 157mg, Vitamin C: 3mg, Calcium: 14mg, Iron: 0.5mg

*with butter
Serves 12
Calories: 144/Calories from fat: 93
Fat: 10.3g, Protein: 3.6 g, Total carb: 8.6g, Fiber: 2g

EGG MUFFINS

SERVES 6 (makes 12; serving size: 2 muffins)

Here is a muffin you don't have to go to the drive-through to get. And unlike anything the drive-through offers, it starts your morning off with a veggie blast! Make them ahead of time so you can have a tasty breakfast on the go, and swap in any season vegetables you like to add variety.

Ingredients:

- 1½ cups grated carrots (from about 4 medium peeled and trimmed carrots)
- ½ cup small diced orange bell peppers
- 9 large eggs
- Salt and pepper, to taste
- 12 tablespoons crumbled feta cheese (¾ cup total)
- Coconut oil or ghee (for coating muffin pan)

Directions:

➤ Preheat oven to 375F. Coat a nonstick 12-cup regular muffin pan *extremely well* with coconut oil or ghee. Be sure to get the base of the cavities and sides, then run your finger over the sides so that every inch is coated or you will be chiseling off stuck food; set pan aside.

➤ In a medium bowl, add carrots, peppers, and toss to combine.

➤ Loosely pile about 2 tablespoons of vegetable mixture in to each muffin cavity, or enough so that each is filled to about ⅔ to ¾ full; equally distribute filling mixture among cavities until gone; set pan aside.

➤ In a 2-cup glass measuring cup (the measuring cup makes for easy pouring), crack the eggs and lightly beat with a whisk. Add the salt and pepper, to taste, and whisk to combine.

continues

Calories: 180/Calories from fat: 97
Fat: 10.8g, Protein: 12.5g, Total carb: 8.2g, Fiber: 1.7g, Sugars: 5g, Sodium: 478mg, Vitamin A: 4917mg, Vitamin C: 20mg, Calcium: 138mg, Iron: 1.5mg

EGG MUFFINS *continued*

➤ Pour about 2-3 tablespoons of egg into each cavity, equally distributing among the cavities. They will be about ¾ full after being topped off with egg.

➤ Top each cup with a generous pinch of cheese, about 1 tablespoon each.

➤ Bake for about 18 to 20 minutes, or until muffins are set, cooked through, and are lightly golden. They will puff in the oven, but sink upon cooling. Allow muffins to cool in pan on top of a wire rack for about 10 minutes before removing.

➤ You will likely need to rim each cavity with a small knife to help dislodge muffins. Muffins will keep airtight for up to 1 week in the fridge.

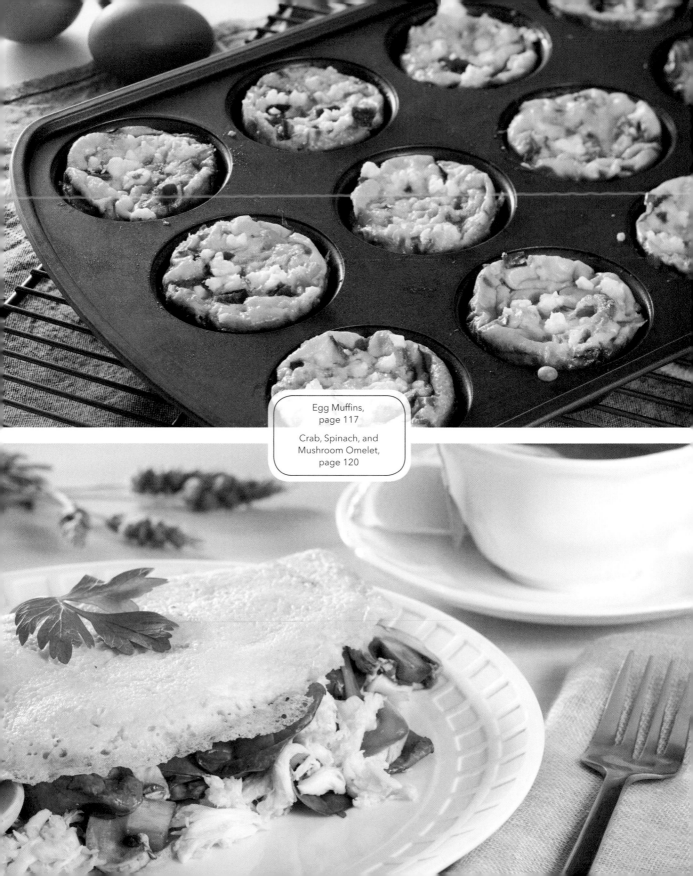

Egg Muffins,
page 117

Crab, Spinach, and
Mushroom Omelet,
page 120

CRAB, SPINACH, AND MUSHROOM OMELET

SERVES 1

The perfect destination for leftover crab from dinner, or reason enough to go out and buy a helping of lump crab meat. This omelet can also be made with lobster meat for a special treat. Be aware that if you swap another fat for the ghee, the nutritional profile will change.

Ingredients:

2 large eggs
¼ cup lump crab meat, shells picked out
1 cup packed baby spinach
¼ cup white button or crimini mushrooms
1 teaspoon ghee
½ tablespoon chopped fresh flat-leaf parsley
Pinch of salt

Directions:

➤ In a small bowl, crack eggs, add a pinch of salt, and whisk.

➤ Heat a 10-inch nonstick skillet to medium-high and melt ghee. Pour the eggs into the pan and cook until the edges are cooked and firm.

➤ Add mushrooms, spinach, and crab to half of the eggs in skillet. Use a fish spatula to gently fold over the other half egg to make a half circle.

➤ Let omelet cook another minute, flip it over, and cook on the other side. You can lift up the top to make sure the egg is no longer runny and cooked through.

➤ Remove to serving plate and sprinkle parsley on top.

Calories: 212/Calories from fat: 125
Fat: 13.9g, Protein: 17.9g, Total carb: 3.1g, Fiber: 0.2g, Sugars: 0.5g, Sodium: 344mg, Vitamin A: 901mg, Vitamin C: 4mg, Calcium: 73mg, Iron: 1.8mg

PORTOBELLO POACHED EGGS

SERVES 4 (serving size: 1 mushroom, 2 eggs, and 1 tablespoon cheese)

Roast meaty Portobello mushrooms and not only will you concentrate their flavor, you'll also make a fun and tasty little holder for poached eggs. The result is a substantial breakfast dish with just the right amount of added cheesy flavor. Try garnishing your eggs with chives, parsley, or thyme.

Ingredients:

8 large eggs
4 Portobello mushrooms,
   cleaned, stems removed
2 teaspoons olive oil
¼ cup goat cheese
¼ teaspoon Himalayan salt
¼ teaspoon fresh ground pepper

Directions:

➤ Preheat oven to 450 degrees.

➤ Place mushrooms gill-side-up on baking sheet, drizzle with olive oil and salt and pepper. Bake for 15 minutes.

➤ Meanwhile, fill a large high-sided skillet with a couple inches of water. Heat the water on high until it reaches a bare simmer and bubbles start appearing at the bottom of the pan, or bring the water to a boil and then lower the heat until the water is at a bare simmer (just a few bubbles coming up now and then).

continues

Calories: 211/Calories from fat: 126
Fat: 14.1g, Protein: 16g, Total carb: 5.5g, Fiber: 1.1g, Sugars: 2g, Sodium: 257mg, Vitamin A: 725mg, Vitamin C: 0mg, Calcium: 107mg, Iron: 1.9mg

PORTOBELLO POACHED EGGS *continued*

➤ Working with the eggs one at a time, crack the egg into a small bowl or cup. Place the bowl close to the surface of the hot water and gently slip the egg into the water. If you want, use a spoon to push some of the egg whites closer to their yolks, to help them hold together. Add all of the eggs you are poaching to the pan in the same way, keeping some distance between them.

➤ Turn off the heat and cover the pan. Set a timer for 3½ minutes. At this point, the egg whites should be completely cooked, while the egg yolks are still runny. Note that the timing depends on the size of the eggs, and if you are cooking at altitude, so adjust accordingly. If you are at altitude, or want firmer egg yolks, you may need to cook them longer.

➤ When the Portobellos are done, remove from the oven and place gill-side-up on serving plates. Sprinkle each mushroom with 1 tablespoon of goat cheese.

➤ Gently lift the poached eggs out of the pan with a slotted spoon and place on top of the prepared mushrooms. Season with pepper to taste. Serve immediately.

 TIP: Grow a window herb garden so you'll always have small amounts of herbs ready for clipping.

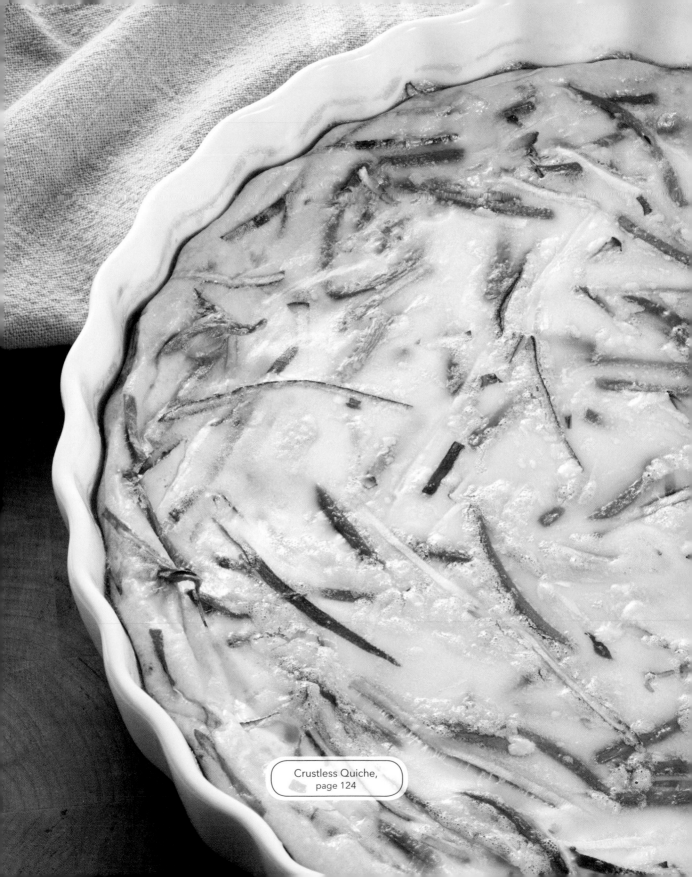

Crustless Quiche,
page 124

CRUSTLESS QUICHE

SERVES 4 (serving size: 3 squares)

This is so flavorful you won't miss the crust—and as a bonus, this quiche will be a cinch to pull off and a guiltless part of an unprocessed diet. It's terrific as leftovers, too; serve them at room temperature or reheat in the oven (not in the microwave, as microwaving will make it rubbery).

Ingredients:

- 1 large zucchini, shredded or grated and strained
- 2 large carrots, peeled, shredded or grated
- ½ teaspoon dried rosemary
- ½ teaspoon dried sage
- ½ teaspoon Himalayan salt
- 12 eggs, beaten
- 1 tablespoon organic, grass-fed butter or ghee

Directions:

➤ Preheat oven to 375 degrees.
➤ Place the grated zucchini in a clean dish towel and wring out the extra water.
➤ Mix together the zucchini, carrots, rosemary, sage and salt and eggs in a large bowl, and then set aside.
➤ Grease a 9x13-inch baking dish with butter, and pour the egg mixture into the pan. Using a fork, swirl sections of the mixture for a swirly pattern.
➤ Bake until the middle is set and edges are golden brown, about 35 minutes. The quiche will puff up while baking and then deflate when removed from the oven. Let cool slightly, then cut into 12 slices and serve warm or at room temperature.

TIP: Try subbing in an equal amount of other vegetables—anything from the crisper drawer that calls out to you.

Calories: 277/Calories from fat: 150
Fat: 16.6g, Protein: 20.1g, Total carb: 11.9g, Fiber: 2.6g, Sugars: 6g, Sodium: 440mg, Vitamin A: 5448mg, Vitamin C: 24mg, Calcium: 96mg, Iron: 2.9mg

9
SNACKS

CRISPY CRACKERS

DAY
4
SNACK

SERVES 10; Serving size: 5 crackers (**MAKES: 50** crackers)

If you ever thought you couldn't make your own crackers, think again. These are super-easy to pull off, even for beginner cooks. Flax seed and egg helps hold them together, no need for the "glue" in gluten required.

Ingredients:

½ cup ground almond meal
  (see note)
½ cup ground flax meal
2 tablespoons shelled hemp
  seeds
1 tablespoon coconut flour
1 large egg
2 tablespoons grass-fed unsalted
  butter, melted
¼ teaspoon Himalayan salt

Directions:

➤ Preheat oven to 300 degrees.

➤ In a large bowl, mix almond meal, flax meal, hemp seeds, coconut flour, and salt together. Pour melted butter and egg over dry mix and combine until dough comes together in a ball.

➤ Roll the dough ball out between two pieces of parchment paper to form a thin sheet (about ¹⁄₁₆" thick). Using a good knife, cut the dough into 1½-inch squares. Reroll dough once or twice to get 50 squares.

➤ Place on baking sheet and bake for 25 to 30 minutes until crisp and dry.

TO make almond meal: take 2 cups almonds place in Vitamix, blender or coffee grinder. Pulse until almonds are broken up to more of a powder. *Do not over mix or you will have almond butter.* Measure out your ⅓ cup for this recipe, store the rest in an air-tight container in the refrigerator or freezer for up to 6 months.

TIP: If your rolled-out dough has ragged edges, no worries—either reroll the scraps and make more crackers, or bake them as is, rustic style. They might not look perfect, but your taste buds won't know the difference.

Calories: 102/Calories from fat: 76
Fat: 8.5g, Protein: 4g, Total carb: 3.4g, Fiber: 2.5g, Sugars: 0g, Sodium: 66mg, Vitamin A: 101mg, Vitamin C: 0mg, Calcium: 28mg, Iron: 0.8mg

FIGS AND RICOTTA

SERVES 4

An elegant looking, luxurious snack that hits the trifecta of creamy, sweet, and crunchy in every bite. Perfect for impromptu entertaining. Bonus: Figs are a wonderful source of antioxidants and vitamins, and they naturally satisfy that craving for sweetness on an unprocessed diet.

Ingredients:

- 4 figs, fresh such as Mission or Turkey
- ¼ cup organic ricotta cheese
- 1 tablespoon chopped pistachios (shelled and unsalted)

Directions:

➤ Cut 2 slits forming an "X" 3 quarters of the way down each fig. Spoon in the ricotta cheese to the "pockets" in the figs. Top with pistachio. Repeat with remaining figs.

Calories: 75/Calories from fat: 27
Fat: 3g, Protein: 2.5g, Total carb: 10.6g, Fiber: 1.6g, Sugars: 8g, Sodium: 24mg, Vitamin A: 140mg, Vitamin C: 1mg, Calcium: 52mg, Iron: 0.3mg

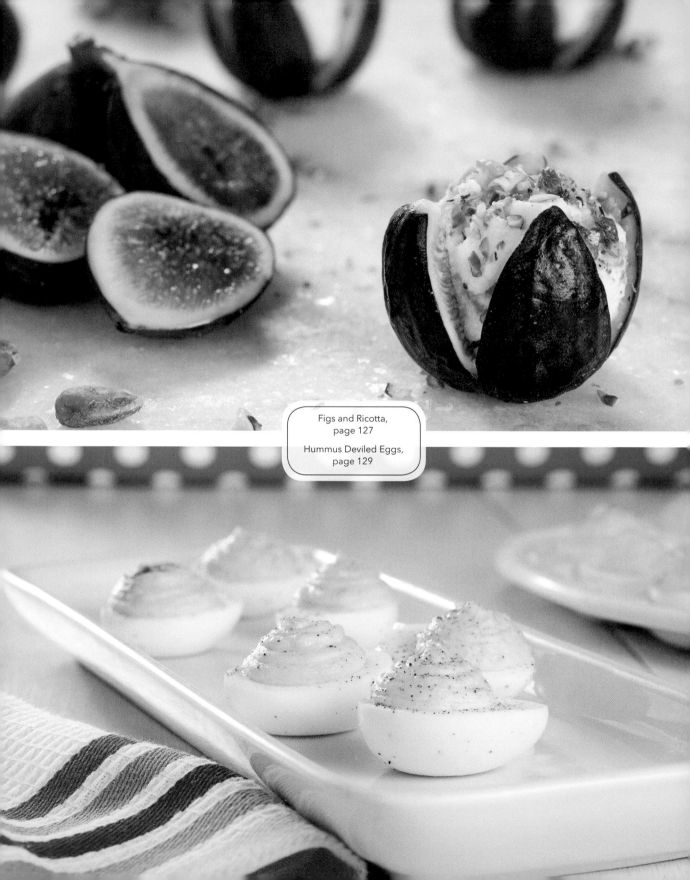

Figs and Ricotta,
page 127

Hummus Deviled Eggs,
page 129

HUMMUS DEVILED EGGS

SERVES 10; **MAKES 20** deviled egg halves

A totally different take on hummus and a clever way of making deviled eggs—with chickpeas blended with the yolks. Chickpeas add a protein boost and a silky smooth texture to your deviled egg filling.

Ingredients:

10 large eggs
1 15-ounce can chickpeas, rinsed and drained
1 clove garlic, peeled, chopped
2-3 tablespoons fresh lemon juice
1 teaspoon coconut aminos
3 tablespoons vegetable broth
⅛ teaspoon paprika for garnish
¼ teaspoon Himalayan salt for garnish

Directions:

➤ Prepare a bowl of ice water and keep cool.

➤ Put eggs in a medium-size saucepan and cover with water by 2 inches. Bring to a boil over high heat (about 13 minutes). Turn off the heat and let sit for 14 minutes. Remove eggs with a slotted spoon and plunge into a bowl of ice water. Cool eggs for 10 minutes. Remove shells when cool. Cut in half lengthwise and scoop out the yolk and reserve in bowl. Repeat with the remaining eggs.

➤ In a blender or food processor (or with a lot of arm power!), combine yolk, chickpeas, garlic, lemon juice, coconut aminos, and vegetable broth until a thick paste forms.

➤ Put the yolk mixture in a piping bag or use a spoon. Pipe or spoon in the yoke hole with hummus mixture and sprinkle with paprika and salt if you choose.

COCONUT AMINOS: A GLUTEN-FREE ALTERNATIVE TO SOY SAUCE

COCONUT aminos are made from the sap of the coconut tree and are similar in taste to soy sauce. But unlike soy sauce, they are gluten-free and soy-free as well. Use them anywhere you'd use soy sauce.

Calories: 108/Calories from fat: 48
Fat: 5.3g, Protein: 7.8g, Total carb: 7.3g, Fiber: 0.1g, Sugars: 0g, Sodium: 179mg, Vitamin A: 320mg, Vitamin C: 2mg, Calcium: 32mg, Iron: 1mg

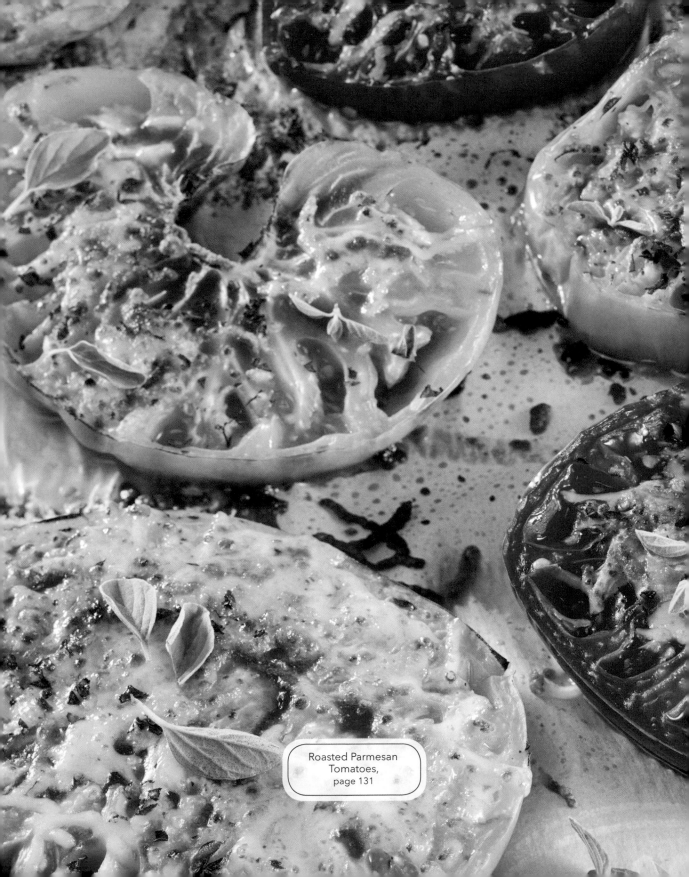

Roasted Parmesan
Tomatoes,
page 131

ROASTED PARMESAN TOMATOES

SERVES 6

Roasting brings out the natural sweetness in tomatoes and concentrates their flavor. Use the cheese sparingly, as a little goes a long way in the flavor department. Perfect as a side to any main dish, or even alongside scrambled eggs for breakfast.

Ingredients:

- 2 beefsteak tomatoes, sliced (4½" thick slices on each tomato)
- 2 tablespoons fresh parmesan cheese, shredded
- 2 teaspoons oregano, fresh or dried
- 1 tablespoon olive oil
- ¼ teaspoon black pepper

Directions:

➤ Preheat oven to 425 degrees. Cover a baking pan or cookie sheet with parchment paper. Thickly slice the tomatoes and place them in a single layer on the prepared pan.

➤ In a small bowl, make a paste by combining the parmesan cheese, 2 tablespoons olive oil, and chopped oregano. Season paste with a few shakes of black pepper.

➤ Spread the paste evenly over each tomato. Bake for 15 minutes until the tops are golden brown and bubbling.

Calories: 58/Calories from fat: 29
Fat: 3.2g, Protein: 2.4g, Total carb: 6g, Fiber: 1.8g, Sugars: 4g, Sodium: 49mg, Vitamin A: 1260mg, Vitamin C: 21mg, Calcium: 51mg, Iron: 0.4mg

CHICKPEA SNACK BARS

YIELD: 24 bars

These protein-packed bars turn chickpeas into a sweet and savory portable snack. Flax seeds really pack in the fiber, and crunchy cacao nibs—made from unsweetened ground-up cacao beans—give an element of chocolaty goodness without the added sugar found in regular chocolate chips.

Ingredients:

- 1½ cups unsalted garbanzo beans, rinsed and drained
- 1 cup almond butter, 16 tablespoons
- 2 cups dried figs, presoaked for an hour
- 1 teaspoon pure vanilla extract
- ¼ teaspoon Himalayan salt
- 1½ cup ground flax seed
- 1 cup cocoa nibs (optional)

Directions:

➤ In a food processor, Vitamix, or blender, mix garbanzo beans, almond butter, figs, vanilla extract, and salt until well blended and smooth.

➤ Add the ground flax seeds and optional cocoa nibs and pulse until they are just mixed in.

➤ Line a 9x13-inch pan with parchment paper and press your mixture into pan all the way to the sides. Refrigerate at least 1 hour before slicing into 24 bars.

➤ Store refrigerated in an airtight container for up to 1 week.

 TIP: You can use a high-speed or regular blender, but a food processor works best

SERVING SIZE: 1 BAR

(TOTALS DO NOT INCLUDE COCOA NIBS.)

Calories: 154/Calories from fat: 80
Fat: 8.8g, Protein: 5.1g, Total carb: 15.5g, Fiber: 4.5g, Sugars: 7g, Sodium: 58mg, Vitamin A: 5mg, Vitamin C: 0mg, Calcium: 65mg, Iron: 1.2mg

VEGGIE SPRING ROLLS

SERVES 6

Lettuce is the unprocessed eater's answer to wrapping, rolling, or stuffing. These veggie-packed lettuce leaf rolls are beautiful to look at and perfect to serve when entertaining. Feel free to swap in any of your favorite vegetables.

Ingredients:

- ½ cup chopped, cooked asparagus
- ½ cup chopped celery
- ½ cup shredded carrots
- 1 avocado, cut lengthwise into slices
- 1 clove garlic, minced
- 1 cup chickpeas, rinsed and drained
- 1 shallot, diced
- 1 teaspoon coconut aminos
- ¼ teaspoon Himalayan salt
- ¼ teaspoon fresh ground black pepper
- 12 pieces of butter lettuce or green leaf lettuce

Directions:

- ➤ In medium bowl, mix all ingredients, except avocado, until combined. Salt and pepper to taste.
- ➤ Distribute 2-3 avocado slices in each lettuce leaf. Spoon filling onto each lettuce leaf, roll up, and serve.

Calories: 126/Calories from fat: 55
Fat: 6.1g, Protein: 4.1g, Total carb: 16g, Fiber: 6.1g, Sugars: 2g, Sodium: 234mg, Vitamin A: 5289mg, Vitamin C: 13mg, Calcium: 42mg, Iron: 1.3mg

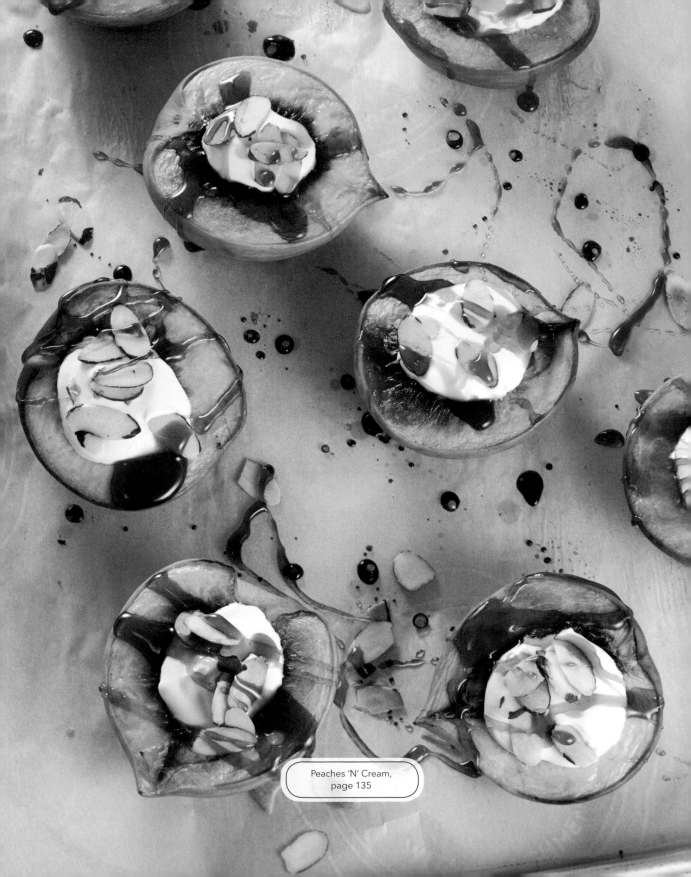

Peaches 'N' Cream,
page 135

PEACHES 'N' CREAM

SERVES 2

Ripe peaches are even juicier after a short stint in the oven, and when you fill them with whole milk, you've got an unprocessed take on classic peaches and cream if you're craving a sweet afternoon snack. You can also make this treat with ripe plums or nectarines.

Ingredients:

- 1 ripe peach, halved with pit removed
- 1 teaspoon coconut oil
- Plain Greek yogurt (Whole or 2%)
- 2 teaspoons sliced almonds

Directions:

➤ Preheat oven to 375.
➤ Place peach halves in an 8"-square 2-quart container. Drizzle coconut oil on top of peach halves and bake until they are heated through but still hold their shape, about 15 minutes. Remove from oven and plate. Scoop Greek yogurt on top and sprinkle on sliced almonds.

Calories: 111/Calories from fat: 58
Fat: 6.6g, Protein: 3.3g, Total carb: 11.1g, Fiber: 1.8g, Sugars: 9g, Sodium: 8mg, Vitamin A: 347mg, Vitamin C: 7mg, Calcium: 37mg, Iron: 0.4mg

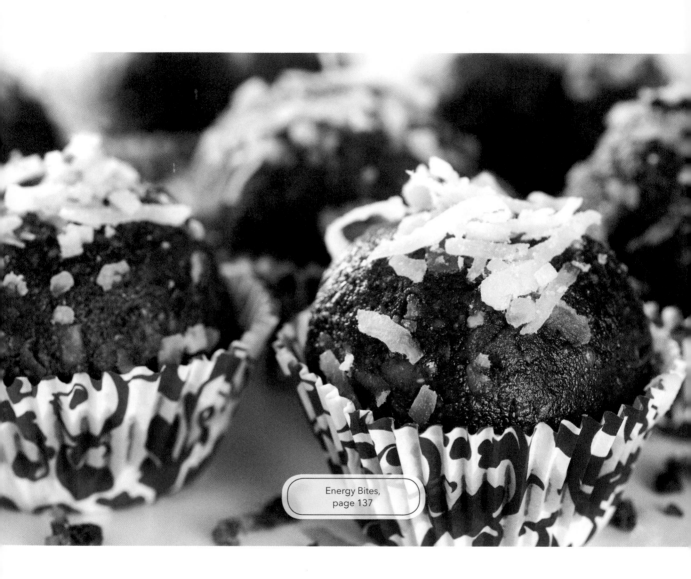

Energy Bites,
page 137

ENERGY BITES

SERVES 10

A protein-packed snack for those days when you need a little extra energy boost without the processed ingredients and shoddy oils you'll find in most supermarket protein snacks. And they taste better than any packaged brand on the market.

Ingredients:

- ⅓ cup almond meal (see note)
- ⅓ cup unsweetened shredded coconut
- 1 tablespoon ground flax seed
- ½ cup almond butter
- ¼ cup cacao powder
- 1 tablespoon chia seeds
- 1 tablespoon agave nectar

Directions:

➤ In a medium-size bowl, combine almond meal, shredded coconut, flax seeds, almond butter, agave nectar, and chia seeds. Mix well until blended. Form into balls, roll in cacao powder, and refrigerate until firm, about 1 hour.

➤ Optional: Top with coconut flakes.

TIP: When you're working out hard, add chia seeds to water or a no-sugar-added beverage—about 1 tablespoon per cup of liquid—and soak for 5 to 10 minutes. The chia seeds will expand and increase hydration, creating an instant sports drink.

TO make almond meal: take 2 cups almonds, place in Vitamix, blender, or coffee grinder. Pulse until almonds are broken up to more of a powder. *Do not over mix or you will have almond butter.* Measure out your ⅓ cup for this recipe, and store the rest in an airtight container in the refrigerator or freezer for up to 6 months.

Calories: 164/Calories from fat: 109
Fat: 12.1g, Protein: 5.6g, Total carb: 8.6g, Fiber: 4.5g, Sugars: 3g, Sodium: 6mg, Vitamin A: 1mg, Vitamin C: 0mg, Calcium: 43mg, Iron: 0.8mg

BOWL FULL OF GOODNESS

SERVES 2

Sweet mango, tart berries, and creamy yogurt, topped with crunchy chia seeds—that, to me, is pure goodness. Chia seeds are a superfood filled with antioxidants and omega-3 fatty acids, and they're a great source of vegetarian protein. The best thing about chia seeds is that most of their carbs come from good-for-you fiber, making them a perfect Jump Start companion! Enjoy a bowlful for breakfast or dessert too!

Ingredients:

- ½ cup ripe mango, peeled, pitted and cut into cubes
- ½ cup blueberries (or other berries of your choice)
- ¼ cup plain Greek yogurt
- 2 tablespoons unsweetened coconut flakes
- 1 teaspoon chia seeds

Directions:

➤ Place fruit in a bowl, and top with yogurt, coconut flakes, and chia seeds in that order.

 TIP: Sprinkle tiny chia seeds over any breakfast, salad, or entree for added protein and a pleasant little crunch.

Calories: 136/Calories from fat: 67
Fat: 7.4g, Protein: 2.8g, Total carb: 15.3g, Fiber: 2.6g, Sugars: 6g, Sodium: 10mg, Vitamin A: 851mg, Vitamin C: 7mg, Calcium: 38mg, Iron: 0.4mg

10

SALADS

AND

SOUPS

LIME-CILANTRO SALAD

SERVES 6 (serving size: about 2 cups)

This crunchy, lettuce-less salad is a perfect make-ahead meal, as sturdy cabbage, cucumber, and carrots will keep for a couple of days in the fridge without losing their shape. Dress and top with the avocado just before serving. The flavors are Asian-inspired and pair perfectly for a crisp, refreshing entrée.

Ingredients:

- 1 head napa cabbage, shredded
- 1 head red cabbage, shredded
- 1 large seedless cucumber, Julienned
- 1 10-ounce bag frozen shelled edamame, thawed
- 2 medium carrots peeled and grated
- 2 green onions, thinly sliced
- 1 avocado, thinly sliced

LIME-CILANTRO DRESSING

Ingredients:

- 1 cup olive oil
- ¾ cup fresh chopped cilantro
- ½ cup coconut nectar
- 1 clove garlic
- Juice of 1 lime
- ½ teaspoon Himalayan salt
- ¼ teaspoon fresh ground pepper

Directions:

➤ In a large salad bowl, toss both cabbages, cucumber, edamame, carrots, and green onions. Set aside.

➤ In a blender, place the olive oil, cilantro, coconut nectar, garlic, lime juice, salt, and pepper.

➤ Blend until smooth.

➤ You can serve salad with dressing already tossed in, with sliced avocado on top. Or place salad on serving plates or bowls and pour salad dressing on top, then the sliced avocados.

TIP: Keep a bag of frozen edamame—fresh soybeans—in your freezer to add as a protein to any vegetable salad. Or look for them fresh in the pod at your local farmers' market in season; to prepare them, boil in salted water for 5 minutes, drain, and pop the beans out of their pods.

Calories: 385/Calories from fat: 286
Fat: 32.1g, Protein: 9.2g, Total carb: 20.6g, Fiber: 10.3g, Sugars: 7g, Sodium: 169mg, Vitamin A: 2325mg, Vitamin C: 59mg, Calcium: 117mg, Iron: 2.3mg

Dressing
Calories: 167/Calories from fat: 161
Fat: 18.2g, Protein: 0.1g, Total carb: 1.8g, Fiber: 0.2g, Sugars: 1g, Sodium: 130mg, Vitamin A: 63mg, Vitamin C: 2mg, Calcium: 3mg, Iron: 0.1mg

ASIAN SALAD

SERVES 4

Veggies, protein, and a small amount of noodles (optional) makes this salad light yet filling, kicking things up a notch with your favorite natural hot sauce for some added heat. A perfect summer dinner, with enough left over to take with you for lunch. The Jump Start meal has none of the optional noodles.

Ingredients:

2 cups shredded chicken
4 cups shredded romaine lettuce
1 cup sliced bell peppers
1 cup julienned seedless cucumber
1 cup sliced celery
1 cup chopped cilantro
3 green onions, sliced
8 ounces rice or pad thai noodles (optional—Not a JS meal with the noodles)
⅓ cup unseasoned rice vinegar
⅓ cup olive oil
1 tablespoon toasted sesame oil
Add your favorite 'natural' hot sauce for desired heat
½ teaspoon Himalayan salt
½ teaspoon ground black pepper

Directions:

➤ For the shredded chicken, you can either purchase a ready-to-eat roasted chicken, preferably organic and without any sauces or marinades added to it, or you can cook it yourself.

➤ To poach: Place raw chicken (2 8-ounce boneless, skinless chicken breasts) and 1 teaspoon salt in a medium saucepan and cover completely with water. Bring to a bare simmer over medium heat until chicken is cooked through, about 20 minutes. Drain chicken, let cool to room temperature, and then refrigerate in an airtight container until ready to use.

➤ If adding noodles, cook according to package instructions, or bring water to a boil (about 17 minutes), add noodles, stir and cover pot. Let sit in hot water 8 to 10 minutes. Then transfer to a bowl of cold water until ready to use, which will keep them from sticking together.

➤ In a large bowl, whisk together vinegar, oil, hot sauce (optional), and sesame oil. Add the chicken breast, romaine, peppers, cucumbers, celery, cilantro, and green onions. Drain the noodles and add to the bowl and toss until evenly tossed and well coated with dressing. Season to taste with salt and pepper.

Calories: 319/Calories from fat: 211
Fat: 23.9g, Protein: 19.9g, Total carb: 6.9g, Fiber: 2.9g, Sugars:3.8g, Sodium: 529mg, Vitamin A: 5962mg, Vitamin C: 61mg, Calcium: 51mg, Iron: 1.5mg

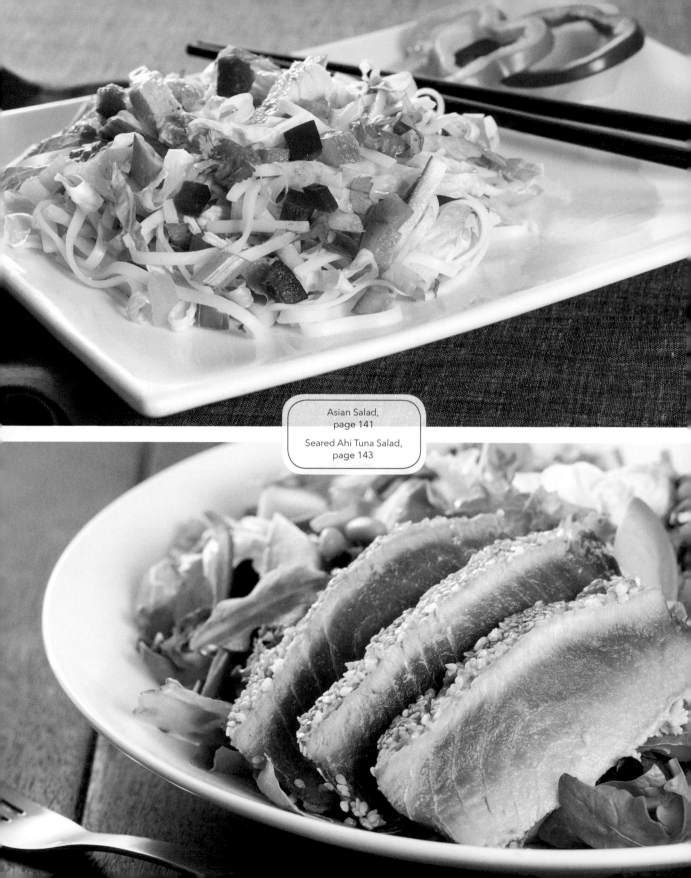

Asian Salad,
page 141

Seared Ahi Tuna Salad,
page 143

SEARED AHI TUNA SALAD

SERVES 4

DAY
2
LUNCH

Wasabi and ginger are a warming, bright-flavored combination, and they cut through the richness of the tuna and avocado to balance out the dish. With tons of veggies to complement the protein- and omega-3-packed tuna, this is a perfect salad from the sea!

Ingredients:

2 8-ounce Ahi tuna steaks
1 teaspoon wasabi paste, separated
3 tablespoons sesame seeds
3 tablespoons olive oil
6 cups mixed dark greens
½ cup shredded carrots
½ cup cucumber, diced
½ cup frozen, thawed, shelled edamame beans
¼ cup cilantro
¼ avocado, sliced
1 tablespoon fresh lime juice
1 teaspoon grated fresh ginger
¼ teaspoon Himalayan salt
Pinch fresh ground black pepper

Directions:

➤ Be sure the tuna is nice and dry on the outside, then rub ½ teaspoon of wasabi paste on both sides of the fish and season with salt and pepper. Place sesame seeds in a shallow dish, then dip the tuna in the sesame seeds on both sides.

➤ Heat a small skillet to medium-high and add 1 tablespoon olive oil. When the oil is hot, lay the tuna in skillet, cook for about 1 minute per side until the outside is seared but the middle is still rare. Be sure not to burn the sesame seeds; if they start to brown too quickly, turn heat down a bit. Remove fish to a plate.

➤ In a small bowl, whisk together lime juice, ginger, remaining ½ teaspoon wasabi, and 2 tablespoons olive oil. Salt and pepper to taste.

➤ In a large salad bowl, toss in lettuce greens, carrots, cucumber, edamame, and cilantro.

➤ Slice the tuna into ¼-inch slices.

➤ Add the lime juice ginger dressing to the salad and toss to coat. Lay the avocado slices on top of salad, and the tuna slices on the very top.

Calories: 285/Calories from fat: 152
Fat: 17.1g, Protein: 26g, Total carb: 8.7g, Fiber: 3.9g, Sugars: 1.9g, Sodium: 225mg, Vitamin A: 6575mg, Vitamin C: 28mg, Calcium: 75mg, Iron: 4.4mg

SUMMERY CHICKEN SALAD

SERVES 6

You'll love the zing of berry flavor and the crunch of the walnuts, and you'll want to make more broth just so you can eat this salad again and again! Or to make things really easy, use the meat from a pre-cooked rotisserie chicken, preferably an organic one.

Ingredients:

2 cups shredded chicken
2 cups fresh trimmed spinach leaves
2 cups fresh spring mix
1 bunch asparagus
2 cups fresh strawberries, sliced
3 tablespoons olive oil, divided
2 tablespoons fresh lemon juice
2 tablespoons balsamic vinegar
½ teaspoon Himalayan salt
¼ teaspoon fresh ground pepper to taste
2 tablespoons toasted walnuts, chopped

Directions:

➤ Preheat oven to 350F.

➤ Prepare asparagus by breaking off the tough ends, cut them into 2-inch pieces. On a baking sheet place asparagus in a single layer and drizzle 1 tablespoon olive oil over top, toss to coat. Season with salt and pepper to taste. Roast asparagus for 15 to 20 minutes until just crisp. Remove from oven when done and let cool.

➤ Using a small bowl, whisk together 2 tablespoons olive oil, lemon juice, agave nectar, and balsamic vinegar. Season with salt and pepper to taste.

➤ In a large salad bowl, combine spinach and spring mix lettuce. Toss to combine the salad greens. Add the asparagus and strawberries and chicken to the dressing, and toss again to thoroughly coat the vegetables with dressing. Divide among 4 bowls and sprinkle with toasted nuts.

 TIP: If strawberries are out of season, raspberries, or another berry, will be equally delicious.

Calories: 395/Calories from fat: 259
Fat: 28.9g, Protein: 24.4g, Total carb: 10g, Fiber: 3.1g, Sugars: 5g, Sodium: 573mg, Vitamin A: 1724 mg, Vitamin C: 49mg, Calcium: 56mg, Iron: 2.5mg

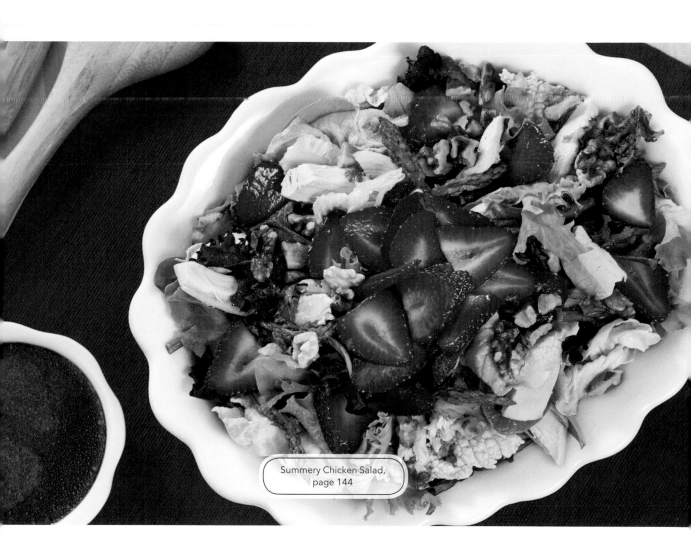
Summery Chicken Salad,
page 144

CHOPPED KALE SALAD

SERVES 8

Kale is so versatile—you can steam it, sauté it, blend it into a smoothie, or make a salad with it. This kale salad is accompanied by carrots, apple, and cabbage, spiced with curry, and sprinkled with pumpkin and pomegranate seeds for texture. Creamy avocado brings it all together. It keeps and travels well, making it great for potlucks and picnics.

Ingredients:

4 cups curly kale leaves, chopped
1 medium carrot, peeled and
   chopped
1 green apple, cored and
   chopped
½ purple cabbage, chopped
1 avocado, cut into cubes
¼ cup raw and hulled pepitas
¼ cup pomegranate seeds
   (optional)
½ lemon, juiced
2 tablespoons red wine vinegar
1 teaspoon curry powder
2 teaspoons agave nectar
½ teaspoon ginger, minced
½ clove garlic, minced
2 tablespoons olive oil
½ teaspoon Himalayan salt
¼ teaspoon fresh ground pepper

Directions:

➤ Prepare the veggies, place the kale in a large bowl, and set the other veggies aside.

➤ Place the lemon juice, red wine vinegar, curry powder, agave nectar, ginger, garlic, and olive oil in a blender and pulse until well combined. Season to taste with salt and pepper.

➤ Add a little bit of the dressing to the bowl with the kale in it. With your hands, massage the dressing in with the kale and let sit for approximately 15 minutes. The acidity from the dressing will help soften the kale a bit.

➤ Put all the veggies in the bowl with the kale, add the dressing, and toss well to combine. When ready to serve, top each with pepitas and pomegranate seeds.

TIP: The secret to successful kale salad is to massage the leaves first to break it down a bit while keeping its characteristic crunch.

Calories: 153/Calories from fat: 85
Fat: 9.5g, Protein: 4.3g, Total carb: 16.9g, Fiber: 5g, Sugars: 7g, Sodium: 143mg, Vitamin A: 4629mg, Vitamin C: 87mg, Calcium: 93mg, Iron: 1.7mg

CHICKEN BROTH

SERVES 14 (serving size: 1 cup)

I prefer homemade stock—and it is really easy to make. You can make a batch or two and keep it on hand in the freezer for when you want to whip up soup.

Ingredients:

- 1 whole chicken, 3½ to 4 lbs, innards removed
- 2 celery stalks with leaves, cut into chunks
- 2 medium carrots, cut into chunks
- 2 medium onions, quartered
- 2 bay leaves
- ½ teaspoon dried rosemary, crushed
- ½ teaspoon dried thyme
- 8 to 10 whole peppercorns
- 1 gallon cold water (or enough water to cover chicken)

Directions:

➤ Place all the ingredients in a soup pot. Slowly bring to a boil over high heat, about 30 minutes; reduce heat. Skim foam. Cover and simmer for 2 hours.

➤ Set chicken aside until cool enough to handle, about 1 hour. Remove meat from bones. Discard bones; save meat for another use. Strain broth, discarding vegetables and seasonings. Refrigerate for 8 hours or overnight. Skim fat from surface.

Calories: 29/Calories from fat: 18
Fat: 2g, Protein: 2.4g, Total carb: 0.3g, Fiber: 0.1g, Sugars: 0g, Sodium: 9.7mg, Vitamin A: 211mg, Vitamin C: 0mg, Calcium: 2mg, Iron: 0.1mg

BUTTERNUT SQUASH SOUP

SERVES 4 (serving size: 1½ cups)

This smooth, velvety, and creamy soup is a wonderful way to welcome in the change of seasons. For variety, try making this recipe with other winter squash varieties such as kabocha, blue hubbard, or red kuri.

Ingredients:

1 medium 2½ lb butternut squash
1 tablespoon olive oil (divided)
1–2 cloves of garlic
½ onion, chopped
4 cups chicken stock (see tip below)
Himalayan salt and fresh ground black pepper

Directions:

➤ Preheat oven to 400 degrees. Line a baking sheet with parchment paper.

➤ Peel and cut squash in ½-inch pieces.

➤ Spread squash onto the prepared baking sheet. Drizzle squash with 1½ teaspoons olive oil, ½ teaspoon salt, and ¼ teaspoon pepper. Toss to combine. Roast until squash is tender, turning once with spatula, about 30 minutes. Heat remaining 1½ teaspoons of oil in a medium saucepan over medium-low heat. Add onion and garlic and cook, stirring occasionally until soft and translucent, about 4 minutes. Add 3 cups of stock and bring to a simmer, about 5 minutes.

➤ Transfer cooked squash to a blender with the stock and puree until smooth. Season to taste with salt and pepper. Serve immediately, or store, refrigerated, in an airtight container for up to 3 days or in the freezer for up to 1 month.

TIP: For homemade chicken stock, see page 147. If you want to make this vegetarian, substitute vegetable for the chicken stock.

Calories: 177/Calories from fat: 50
Fat: 5.6g, Protein: 5.2g, Total carb: 30.7g, Fiber: 5.3g, Sugars: 6g, Sodium: 400mg, Vitamin A: 25528mg, Vitamin C: 52mg, Calcium: 125mg, Iron: 1.9mg

GREEN GAZPACHO

SERVES 3

If you've never eaten a green zebra tomato, you're in for a treat! This tomato is an heirloom variety with gorgeous green and yellow striped skin and a slightly tart, full flavor. The best place to find green zebras is at your neighborhood farmers' market in season. If unavailable, substitute another juicy local tomato—your soup might not be green, but it will be every bit as delicious.

Ingredients:

- 1 lb green zebra tomatoes, cored and chopped
- 1 cucumber unpeeled, seeded and diced
- 1 red onion, diced
- 1 ripe avocado, peeled, pitted, and diced
- 1 jalapeño, seeded and diced
- 3 cloves garlic, chopped
- Juice of 1 lime
- ¼ cup white wine vinegar
- 2 tablespoons cilantro
- 1 tablespoon olive oil
- 1 teaspoon Himalayan salt
- ½ teaspoon fresh ground pepper

Directions:

➤ Separate chopped tomato, cucumber and onion in half.

➤ In blender, add ½ tomato, ½ cucumber, and ½ onion along with the avocado, jalapeño, garlic, lime juice and ¼ cup white wine vinegar. Blend until you have a smooth puree; you might need to add a little cold water if puree is still too chunky.

➤ Place this mixture into a large non-reactive (non-metal) bowl.

➤ In the blender, add other half of the tomato, cucumber, and onion along with cilantro and olive oil. Pulse until you get a chunky puree.

➤ Combine both purees in the bowl and add salt and pepper, mix well.

➤ Cover and refrigerate overnight. The longer it chills the better the flavor will come out.

TIP: Make your gazpacho a day ahead to allow the flavors to develop to their fullest.

Calories: 217/Calories from fat: 131
Fat: 14.7g, Protein: 5g, Total carb: 21.4g, Fiber: 7.9g, Sugars: 10g, Sodium: 533mg, Vitamin A: 1378mg, Vitamin C: 61mg, Calcium: 63mg, Iron: 1.7mg

SPICY EGG DROP SOUP

SERVES 4 (serving size: 1⅓ cups)

This egg drop soup, a healthy take on a classic, has great texture and flavor, but it can be spicy! You might want to cut down on the amount of chilies. Make it with homemade broth to elevate the flavor and nutritional profile of the soup.

Ingredients:

6 cups chicken broth (see recipe on page 147)
1 large carrot, peeled and sliced into half moons
1 clove garlic, minced
⅛ teaspoon fresh ginger, grated
3 Thai chilies, seeded and diced (if you want it less spicy, use fewer chilies)
3 tablespoons coconut aminos
3 large eggs
2 medium green onions, diced
¼ cup fresh cilantro, chopped
Himalayan salt and freshly ground black pepper to taste

Directions:

➤ Bring chicken broth to a boil in a medium-size saucepan over high heat, about 10 minutes.

➤ Add the carrot, garlic, ginger, chilies, and coconut aminos. Turn heat down and simmer until flavors develop and carrot is tender, 15 minutes.

➤ Whisk the eggs in a small bowl. Slowly pour the egg into the soup and stir a few times as you pour.

➤ Remove from heat and add in the green onion and cilantro. Season to taste with salt and pepper.

Calories: 133/Calories from fat: 73
Fat: 8.2g, Protein: 8.7g, Total carb: 5.3g, Fiber: 1.3g, Sugars: 2g, Sodium: 492mg, Vitamin A: 4062mg, Vitamin C: 5mg, Calcium: 32mg, Iron: 1.3mg

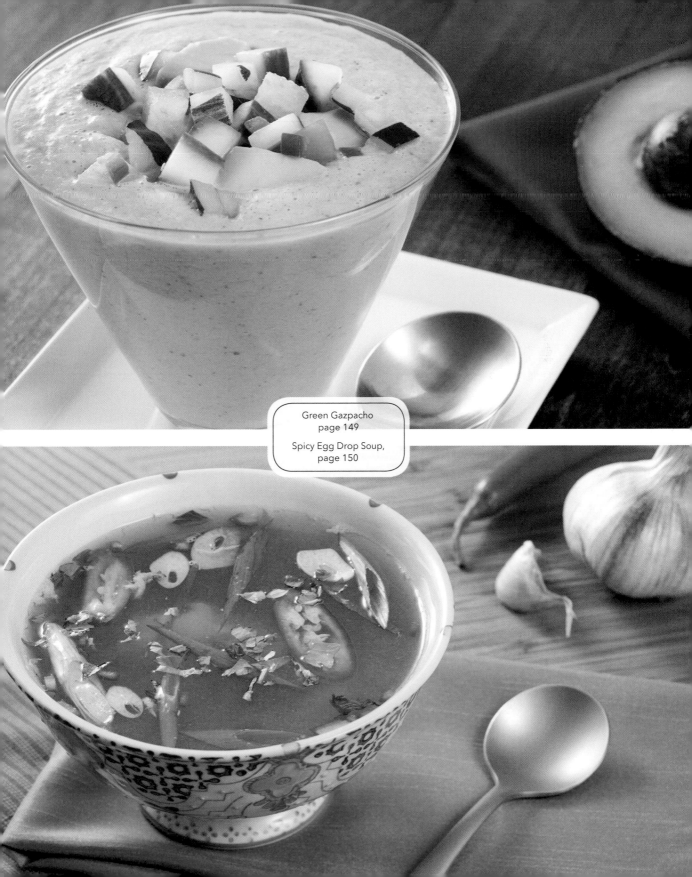

Green Gazpacho
page 149

Spicy Egg Drop Soup,
page 150

HEARTY VEGETABLE SOUP

SERVES 4 (serving size: about 3 cups)

Chock-full of veggie goodness! For a balanced vegetarian meal, add a protein source such as edamame or chickpeas. Or crack an egg or two directly into the soup when it's just about done; cover and cook for a few minutes, until poached to your liking.

Ingredients:

    1 onion, chopped
    2 cloves garlic, minced
    2 carrots, diced
    1 zucchini, diced, medium size
    2 cups broccoli, chopped
    1 cup mushrooms, sliced
    2 cups cauliflower, chopped
    1 bunch fresh spinach, or 2 cups
        fresh baby spinach
    2 cups diced tomatoes (whole
        tomatoes)
    8 cups water
    1 tablespoon coconut oil
    Himalayan salt and fresh ground
        pepper to taste

Directions:

➤ In a large stock pot, heat coconut oil over medium-high heat and sauté onions until translucent, about 3 minutes. Add garlic and sauté another 30 seconds.

➤ Add water, tomatoes, and all vegetables but the spinach. Bring to a boil, about 20 minutes, reduce heat, cover and simmer for 30 minutes, until vegetables are tender. If you want a soup with more broth, add more water.

➤ Stir in spinach and salt and pepper to taste.

 TIP: For non-vegetarians, sub in chicken broth for the water for developed flavor and added nutrients.

Calories: 126/Calories from fat: 37
Fat: 4.2g, Protein: 6g, Total carb: 20.3g, Fiber: 6.4g, Sugars: 10g, Sodium: 475mg, Vitamin A: 4499mg, Vitamin C: 97mg
Calcium: 80mg, Iron: 1.8mg

CHICKEN AVOCADO SOUP

SERVES 4

Wholesome chicken soup made easy, and avocado slices on top are what really give this soup its unique flavor. Swap in any seasonal vegetables you like to change things up.

Ingredients:

½ tablespoon olive oil
2 chicken breasts, bone in, skin on
1 onion chopped
1 clove garlic, minced
3 carrots, peeled and sliced
2 stalks celery, sliced
6 cups water
¼ cup cilantro, chopped
1 ripe avocado peeled, pitted, and sliced
1½ teaspoons Himalayan salt
½ teaspoon fresh ground black pepper

Directions:

➤ Heat the olive oil in a large heavy pot over medium-high heat.

➤ Season chicken with ½ teaspoon salt and ½ teaspoon pepper. Place chicken skin side-down in pot and brown slightly on all sides, about 8 to 10 minutes. Remove chicken to a plate to rest.

➤ Add onion, garlic, carrots, and celery and cook, scraping up brown bits until vegetables begin to soften, about 3 minutes.

➤ Return chicken and juices to the pot and add water. Bring to a boil (14 minutes), reduce to a simmer, and cook until the chicken is very tender, about 45 minutes. Turn off heat.

➤ Remove chicken from pot and let cool until easy to handle, about 15 minutes.

➤ Remove meat from bone and shred, and discard skin. Return meat to pot and stir in cilantro.

➤ Pour soup into 4 bowls and top each with sliced avocado. Serve immediately or refrigerate in an airtight container for up to 4 days or freeze up to 1 month.

Note: you can use ghee instead of the olive oil.

Calories: 254/Calories from fat: 119
Fat: 13.2g, Protein: 19.5g, Total carb: 16g, Fiber: 6.2g, Sugars: 6g, Sodium: 648mg, Vitamin A: 2677mg, Vitamin C: 15mg, Calcium: 46mg, Iron: 1.3mg

CHICKEN AND KALE SOUP

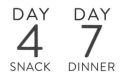

DAY
4
SNACK

DAY
7
DINNER

SERVINGS: 6

Bursting with chunks of kale, veggies, and chicken, this soup will warm you from your head to your toes. If you're out of kale, feel free to swap in spinach.

Ingredients:

4 chicken breasts, bone-in and skin-on
2 onions cut into chunks
6 carrots, trimmed, peeled, and sliced crosswise into ¼" rounds
6 celery stalks, trimmed and sliced crosswise into ¼"-thick slices
8 cups water
2 cloves garlic, sliced
1 bunch kale
1½ teaspoons Himalayan salt
½ teaspoon ground black pepper

Directions:

➤ In a large stock pot, add water, chicken breasts, carrots, celery, onion, garlic, salt, and pepper. Bring to a boil, reduce to a simmer, and cook until chicken is cooked through and veggies are tender, about 15 minutes more.

➤ Remove chicken from pot and let cool until easy to handle, about 15 minutes.

➤ Meanwhile, remove kale from stems and cut into bite-size pieces, add to the chicken soup broth. Stir until wilted. When adding spinach and/or kale, just toss leaves into pot and stir until mixed in with other veggies. Turn off heat.

➤ Remove chicken from bone and skin and shred. Add chicken back to pot, stir to combine.

➤ After adding chicken back in, if you would like some more broth you may add 2 more cups of water. Serve warm or refrigerate in an airtight container for up to 4 days. Freeze for up to 1 month.

Calories: 202/Calories from fat: 32
Fat: 3.5g, Protein: 29g, Total carb: 15.5g, Fiber: 3.6g, Sugars: 4g, Sodium: 504mg, Vitamin A: 1942mg, Vitamin C: 114mg, Calcium: 167mg, Iron: 2.4mg

11
SIDES

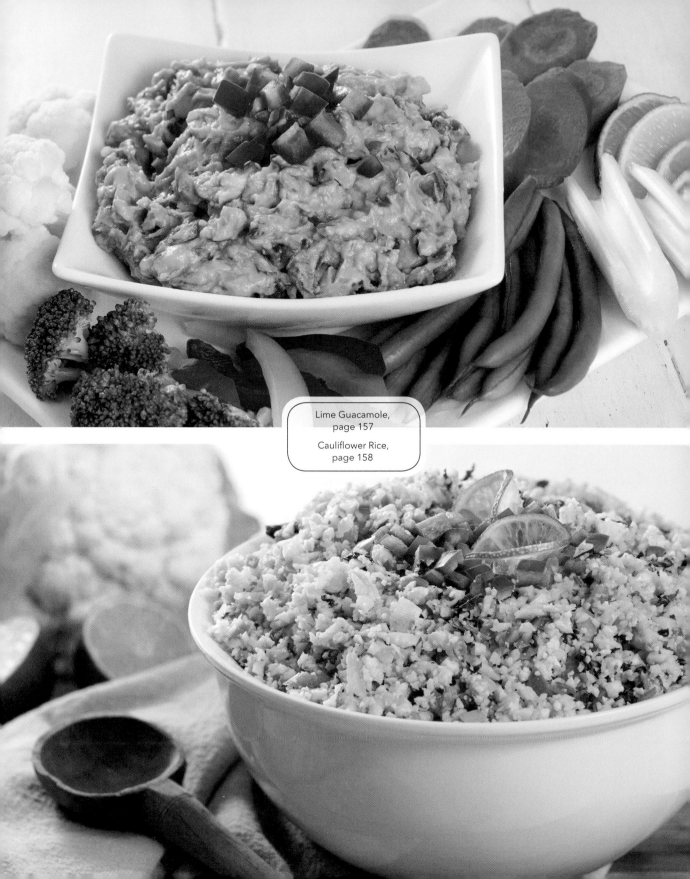

Lime Guacamole,
page 157

Cauliflower Rice,
page 158

LIME GUACAMOLE

SERVES 8

DAY
4
SNACK

DAY
7
DINNER

When you unprocess your diet, you'll have a newfound appreciation for the flavors of real food. So when you hear the word *guacamole,* the first word that comes to your mind won't be *chips* but fresh vegetable sticks! You'll also love this guac spread over a burger or added to a wrap.

Ingredients

  2 ripe avocados, peeled, pitted,
    and diced
  Juice of 1 lime
  2 cloves garlic
  ½ ripe tomato diced
  2 tablespoons chopped cilantro
  ½ teaspoon Himalayan salt
  ¼ teaspoon fresh ground pepper

Directions:

➤ Using a blender or food processor, put in all the ingredients except Himalayan salt and pepper.

➤ Pulse ingredients until blended but still some small chunks, add salt and pepper to taste.

➤ Store in covered container, flavors will come out more as it sits for a little while.

Calories: 96/Calories from fat: 75
Fat: 8.3g, Protein: 1.3g, Total carb: 6.1g, Fiber: 4g, Sugars: 1g, Sodium: 100mg, Vitamin A: 178mg, Vitamin C: 9mg, Calcium: 11mg, Iron: 0.4mg

CAULIFLOWER RICE

SERVES 4

Now you can have your "rice on the side" without busting the carb bank! You'll be amazed at how close you can get your cauliflower to the texture of rice just by pulsing it in the food processor, and you'll love how satisfied it leaves you feeling. Cauliflower is kind of like a blank canvas, soaking in whatever flavors you add to it; lime, cilantro, and tomatoes jazz up our cauliflower rice. If you prefer, this recipe can be made with coconut oil instead of butter.

Ingredients:

1 head cauliflower
1 tablespoon butter
½ yellow onion, chopped
½ jalapeño, seeded and chopped (optional)
Juice and zest of 1 lime
½ cup cilantro, chopped
½ teaspoon Himalayan salt
½ teaspoon pepper
½ cup chopped tomato (optional)

Directions:

➤ Cut the cauliflower into small florets. Pulse in two batches in blender or food processor until cauliflower resembles rice. Cauliflower can also be grated on a cheese grater.

➤ Preheat 1 tablespoon butter or oil in a large high-sided skillet. Cook onion in the pan over medium-high heat, stirring occasionally until onion turns translucent, about 3 minutes.

➤ Add cauliflower and jalapeño to pan, stirring occasionally until warmed through, about 3 minutes. Mix in lime juice and zest, then add the cilantro, stir until well blended. Season to taste with salt and pepper. Top with chopped tomato.

TIP: After you've made this dish a few times, why not try branching out with your own cauliflower rice variations—how about cucumber, dill, and capers or parsley, scallions, and lemon juice for starters?

Calories: 92/Calories from fat: 26
Fat: 3g, Protein: 4.6g, Total carb: 13.9g, Fiber: 4.9g, Sugars: 6g, Sodium: 279mg, Vitamin A: 437mg, Vitamin C: 130mg, Calcium: 52mg, Iron: 0.9mg

NO-POTATO MASHED POTATOES

SERVES 4

Go ahead and indulge in these rich and creamy potatoes. Oh, wait, they aren't potatoes! When you blend cauliflower with garlic and butter, you perform a little magic trick, giving a whole new meaning to the concept of comfort food. Immune-boosting shiitakes are the crowning glory to this spudless classic.

Ingredients:

- 2 heads cauliflower, trimmed, cored, and cut into 2" florets
- 2 cloves garlic
- 2 tablespoons clarified butter
- ½ cup shiitake mushrooms, sliced (about 3 to 4 mushrooms; stems trimmed and sliced)
- 1 teaspoon pink Himalayan rock salt
- ½ teaspoon ground black pepper
- 4 sprigs parsley, chopped (garnish)

Directions:

➤ Line a large saucepan with a steamer basket and 3 to 4 cups of water. Cover the saucepan and bring the water to a boil over high heat. Once boiling, add the cauliflower and garlic to boiling water. Cover and steam until the cauliflower and garlic are tender, about 8 to 10 minutes.

➤ Meanwhile, melt 1 teaspoon ghee in a medium skillet over medium-high heat. Add the mushrooms and cook, stirring a few times, until lightly browned, about 6 minutes.

➤ Place the cauliflower, garlic, remaining butter, salt, and pepper in a food processor, and process until smooth and creamy. You may add any other spices you like. Top with sautéed shiitake mushrooms and parsley.

Calories: 120/Calories from fat: 58
Fat: 6.5g, Protein: 5.2g, Total carb: 13.9g, Fiber: 5.4g, Sugars: 5g, Sodium: 505mg, Vitamin A: 261mg, Vitamin C: 117mg, Calcium: 60mg, Iron: 1.2mg

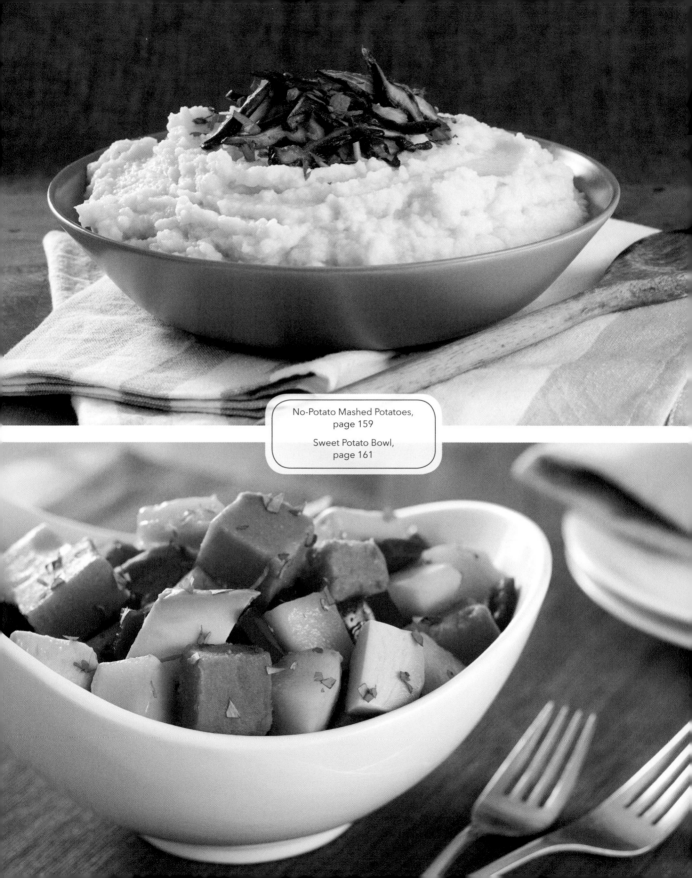

No-Potato Mashed Potatoes,
page 159

Sweet Potato Bowl,
page 161

SWEET POTATO BOWL

SERVES 4

That beautiful orange color? It's thanks to the sweet potato's beta-carotene, a potent anti-oxidant that's converted to vitamin A in the body. Keep the skin on your sweet potatoes, as it contains lots of fiber. It's important to note that the skin is also where the pesticides can concentrate, so go organic if at all possible.

Ingredients:

- 1 large sweet potato
- 1 mango peeled and cut into 1" dice
- 1 red bell pepper, seeded and chopped
- ½ avocado, peeled, seeded, and cut into 1" dice
- ¼ cup cilantro, chopped
- Juice of 1 lime

Directions:

➤ Preheat oven to 400 degrees.

➤ Use the tines of a fork to prick the potato all over. Place potato on a small baking sheet to catch any drips. Place in oven and roast until a knife can easily pierce through the middle of the potato, about 45 minutes. Let potato cool to room temperature, about 30 minutes, or refrigerate until ready to use.

➤ Peel the sweet potato, cut into 1-inch pieces, and place in a medium bowl.

➤ Top with mango, bell pepper, avocado, and cilantro.

➤ Drizzle lime juice over top and toss gently to combine.

Calories: 123/Calories from fat: 3.8
Fat: 0.4g, Protein: 1.8g, Total carb: 28.8g, Fiber: 3.9g, Sugars: 6g, Sodium: 49mg, Vitamin A: 14421mg, Vitamin C: 61mg, Calcium: 30mg, Iron: 0.7mg

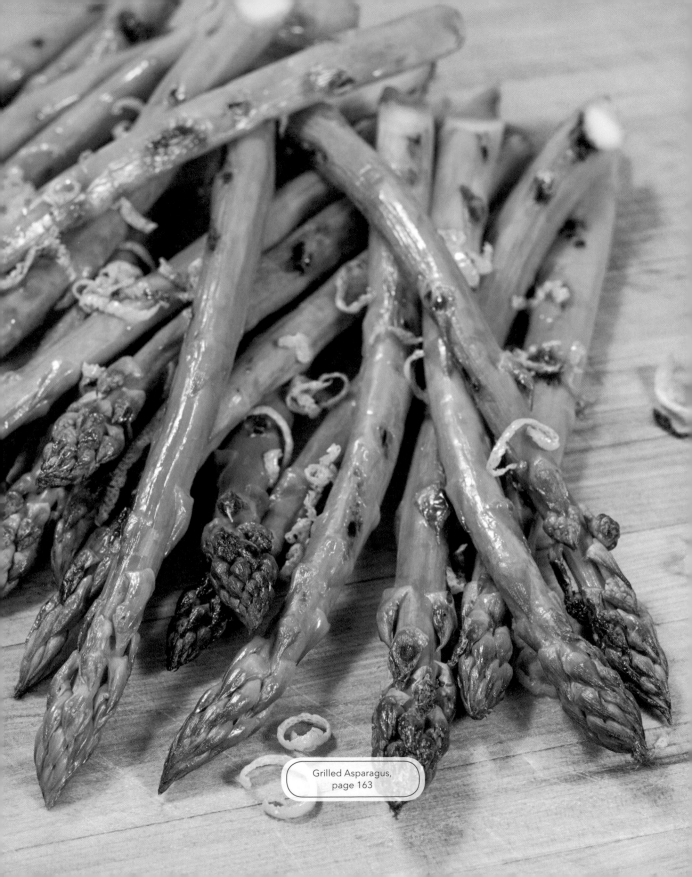

Grilled Asparagus,
page 163

GRILLED ASPARAGUS

SERVES 2

DAY
2
DINNER

DAY
5
DINNER

Grilling makes everything taste great without adding calories, and there's nothing better than grilled asparagus with a fresh squeeze of lemon. If you don't have access to a grill, make yours in a grill pan on the stovetop.

Ingredients:

1 lb fresh asparagus, trimmed
1 tablespoon olive oil
1 tablespoon lemon zest
Juice of ½ lemon
¼ teaspoon Himalayan salt
¼ teaspoon fresh ground black
    pepper to taste

Directions:

➤ Heat grill to medium-high.

➤ Break or cut off the tough end of the asparagus, lay asparagus on baking sheet, and drizzle olive oil and lemon zest over the top. Salt and pepper to taste. Toss the asparagus around in the olive and seasoning until well coated.

➤ While grill is hot, place the asparagus on the grill to cook; you want the asparagus just crisp tender, about 2 to 3 minutes per side. Turn once to get grill marks on the other side.

➤ Remove asparagus to serving plate and sprinkle with the lemon juice. Serve warm or at room temperature.

Calories: 108/Calories from fat: 60
Fat: 6.8g, Protein: 4.4g, Total carb: 10.3g, Fiber: 4.7g, Sugars: 5g, Sodium: 191mg, Vitamin A: 1072mg, Vitamin C: 29mg, Calcium: 49mg, Iron: 1mg

NUTTY BRUSSELS

SERVES 8

Think you aren't a fan of Brussels sprouts? Roasting them will convert you, as it avoids the sulfury smell and mushy texture many of us associate with over-boiled sprouts. Think of them as adorable mini cabbages and you'll come to love them! And if you need more convincing, remember that they are a member of the cruciferous family, known for its potent antioxidant properties.

Ingredients:

- 2 lbs Brussels sprouts, trimmed and halved if large
- 8 raw pecans, chopped
- 2 tablespoons olive oil
- 3 shallots
- 3 cloves garlic, minced
- ¼ teaspoon pink Himalayan salt
- ¼ teaspoon fresh ground black pepper

Directions:

➤ Cut Brussels sprouts in half, place in a gallon-size ziplock bag.

➤ Slice shallots and place in bag with Brussels sprouts. Add olive oil, garlic, salt, and pepper to taste, mix all ingredients until Brussel sprouts are well coated.

➤ Let sit at room temperature for approximately 30 minutes, turning the bag several times.

➤ Place contents of bag on a large baking sheet, spread pecans over the top. Bake at 350 degrees for 30 minutes. Depending on how crunchy you like them, you may want to bake for a longer or shorter time. Check them periodically so you can judge a cooking time that suits your taste buds.

Calories: 137/Calories from fat: 81
Fat: 9g, Protein: 3.6 g, Total carb: 11g, Fiber: 4.1g, Sugars: 3g, Sodium: 123mg, Vitamin A: 452mg, Vitamin C: 82mg, Calcium: 30mg, Iron: 0.4mg

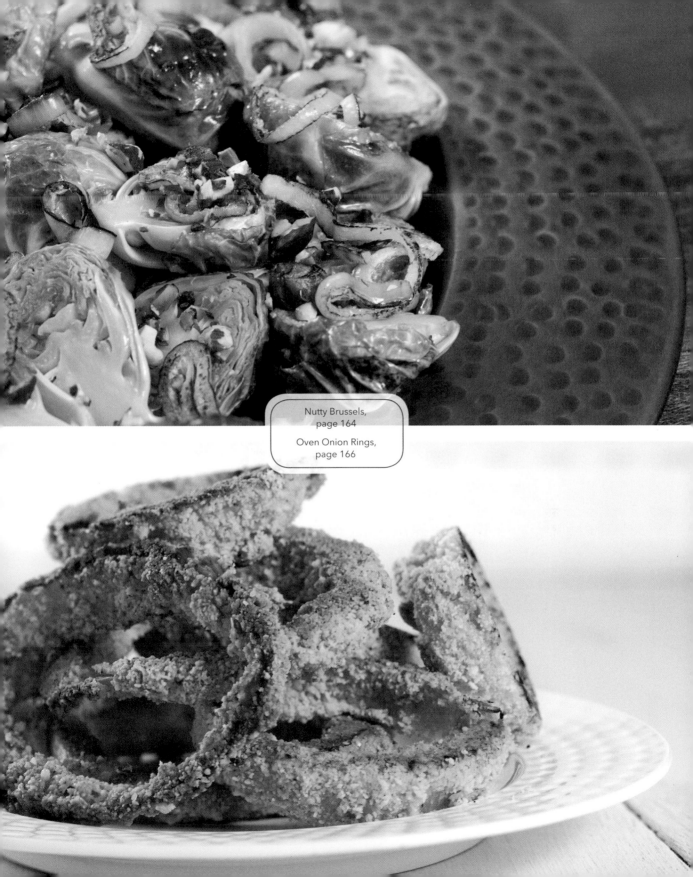

Nutty Brussels,
page 164

Oven Onion Rings,
page 166

OVEN ONION RINGS

SERVES 6

Yes, you read the title right! These onion rings get a Jump Start stamp of approval! Just swap almond flour for traditional wheat flour, ditch the fryer, and bake your rings into sweet, crunchy deliciousness! Pull up a burger and you've just reinvented an all-American classic.

Ingredients:

1 large onion
1½ cups almond flour
¾ teaspoon cayenne
¾ teaspoon garlic salt
¾ teaspoon fresh ground pepper
1 large egg
2 tbsp coconut oil

Directions:

➤ Preheat oven to 400 degrees.

➤ Slice the onion into ½-inch rings and separate.

➤ In a small bowl whisk egg with 1 tablespoon of water.

➤ On a flat plate or shallow dish mix the dry ingredients, almond flour, cayenne, garlic salt, and pepper.

➤ Dip the onion rings individually into the egg, let excess run off. Then place it in the dry mixture coating both sides, shake them off slightly.

➤ Lay all onion rings on a parchment-lined baking sheet. Lightly drizzle coconut oil onto rings, this is so you can have some crispness when baking. You may choose not to bake them with the oil if you prefer.

➤ Bake onion rings for 15 minutes, pull baking sheet out and turn rings over and bake for an additional 15 minutes, until light brown and crispy.

Calories 227/Calories from fat: 180
Fat: 20g, Protein: 7g, Total Carb: 9g, Fiber: 4g, Sugars: 2g, Sodium: 258 mg, Vitamin A 50mg, Vitamin C 1.8mg , Calcium 1.26 mg, Iron 70 mg

CILANTRO SWEETENED SWEET POTATOES

SERVES 8

Earthy sweet potatoes with a hint of lime make a fiber-filled companion for any time you fire up the grill. Sweet potatoes are one of my favorite carb companions for my Jump Start meals.

Ingredients:

>   3 medium sweet potatoes
>   2 tablespoons extra virgin
>   olive oil
>   ½ teaspoon Himalayan salt

CILANTRO LIME DRESSING:

>   ¼ cup finely chopped fresh
>   cilantro
>   1 teaspoon lime zest
>   2 tablespoons fresh lime juice
>   2 tablespoons olive oil

Directions:

➤ Preheat a grill or grill pan to medium heat. Peel the potatoes and slice on a bias crosswise into ¼-inch thick slices. Place the potatoes in a large bowl, drizzle with 2 tablespoons olive oil, and lightly season with salt.

➤ Combine all the dressing ingredients in a small bowl and whisk together.

➤ Lay the sweet potato pieces on the grill (grill in batches if necessary). Cover the grill and cook until each side gets some grill marks, about 6 minutes for each side until tender.

➤ Toss the potatoes in a bowl with the dressing and serve hot.

Calories: 146/Calories from fat: 60
Fat: 6.8g, Protein: 1.6g, Total carb: 20.4g, Fiber: 3.1g, Sugars: 4g, Sodium: 150mg, Vitamin A: 14,113mg, Vitamin C: 5mg, Calcium: 32mg, Iron: 0.7mg

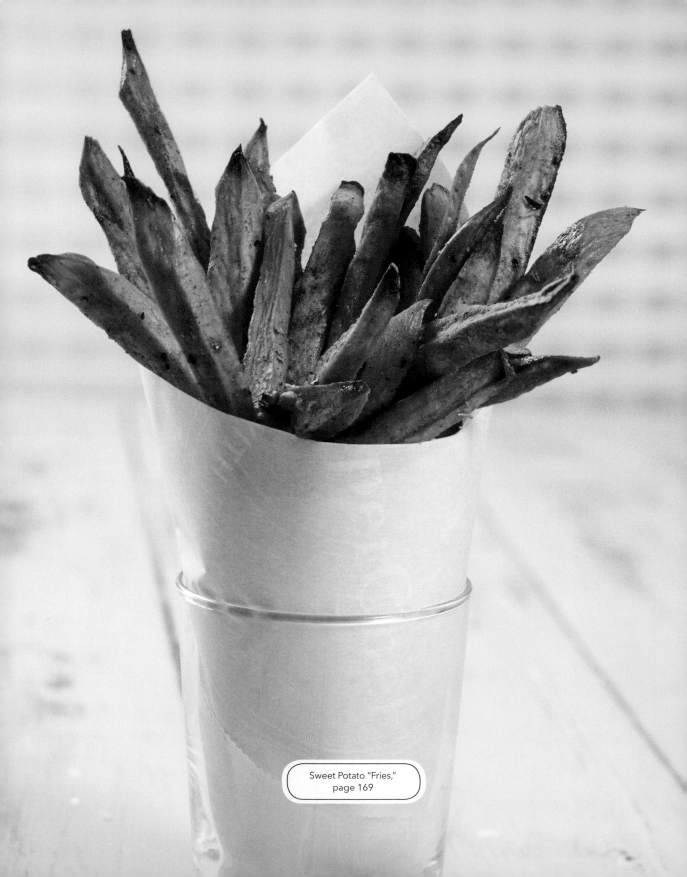

Sweet Potato "Fries,"
page 169

SWEET POTATO "FRIES"

SERVES 8

If you find the idea of giving up a burger and fries as part of an unprocessed diet challenging for you, guess what? You don't have to! Try the burger on page 221, and serve it with these sweet and savory *baked* sweet potato fries. And you'll feel great, not guilty, when you clean your plate!

Ingredients:

2 large sweet potatoes
2 tablespoons olive oil
½ lemon, juiced
2 teaspoons Jamaican seasoning (recipe below)

Spice Ingredients:

1 tablespoon garlic powder
2 teaspoons cayenne pepper
2 teaspoons onion powder
2 teaspoons dried thyme
2 teaspoons dried parsley
2 teaspoons Himalayan salt
1 teaspoon paprika
1 teaspoon ground allspice
½ teaspoon fresh ground black pepper
½ teaspoon dried crushed red pepper
½ teaspoon ground nutmeg
½ teaspoon cinnamon

Combine all ingredients, and store in an airtight container for up to three months.

Directions:

➤ Preheat oven to 400 degrees with racks on the upper and lower thirds. Line two baking sheets with parchment paper and set aside.

➤ Cut sweet potatoes in half lengthwise, then cut each half into ½-inch wedges resembling thick-cut fries. It is okay to make them any size you want, but be sure they aren't too thick or they will take longer to cook.

➤ In a gallon-sized ziptop bag or alternately, in a large bowl, put in potatoes, add olive oil, lemon, and Jamaican seasoning. Shake bag or toss in the bowl until fries look evenly coated with ingredients.

➤ Place fries on the prepared baking sheets, and bake, rotating pans halfway through cooking until tender, depending on size about 40 to 45 minutes.

Calories: 150/Calories from fat: 33
Fat: 3.7g, Protein: 2.4g, Total carb: 27.9g, Fiber: 4.6g, Sugars: 6g, Sodium: 452mg, Vitamin A: 18498mg, Vitamin C: 5mg, Calcium: 52mg, Iron: 1.3mg

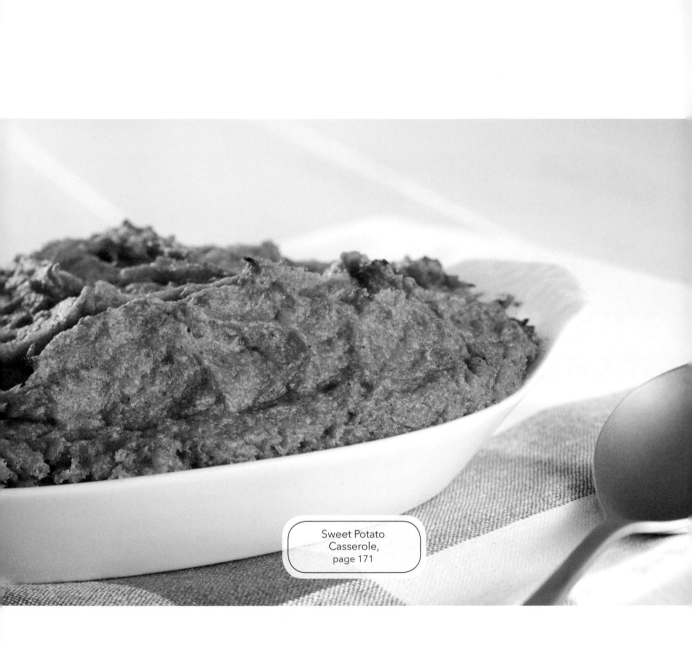

Sweet Potato
Casserole,
page 171

SWEET POTATO CASSEROLE

SERVES 12

Once you've unprocessed your diet, your taste buds come to appreciate the flavor of naturally sweet foods like sweet potatoes. With a little cinnamon and nutmeg sprinkled on top, you won't even think to miss the mini marshmallows!

Ingredients:

- 4.5 lbs sweet potatoes (medium-sized sweet potatoes)
- 3 tablespoons grass-fed organic butter
- ¼ cup fresh squeezed orange juice (whole orange = 1½ ounces) (¼ cup juice = 2 ounces)
- 1 tablespoon pure vanilla extract
- ½ teaspoon ground cinnamon
- ½ teaspoon freshly grated nutmeg
- 1 tablespoon coconut oil, melted for coating baking dish (½ ounce)

Directions:

- ➤ Preheat oven to 400 degrees.
- ➤ Prick potatoes all over with the tines of a fork and place on a baking sheet. Bake until soft when pierced with a knife, about 1 hour 15 minutes. Let cool slightly until easy to handle, about 15 minutes.
- ➤ Remove skins and any potato strings from hot potatoes using a dish cloth and a paring knife. Use a potato masher or ricer to mash well.
- ➤ Add all ingredients to potatoes and mix well.
- ➤ Coat 9x13-inch baking dish lightly with coconut oil and add the mashed sweet potatoes. You can sprinkle some additional cinnamon on top if desired.
- ➤ Reduce oven temperature to 350 degrees and bake until flavors come together, about 15-20 minutes. It will depend on preferred doneness.

Calories: 188/Calories from fat: 37
Fat: 4.2g, Protein: 2.8g, Total carb: 35g, Fiber: 5.2g, Sugars: 8g, Sodium: 119mg, Vitamin A: 24231mg, Vitamin C: 7mg, Calcium: 54mg, Iron: 1.1mg

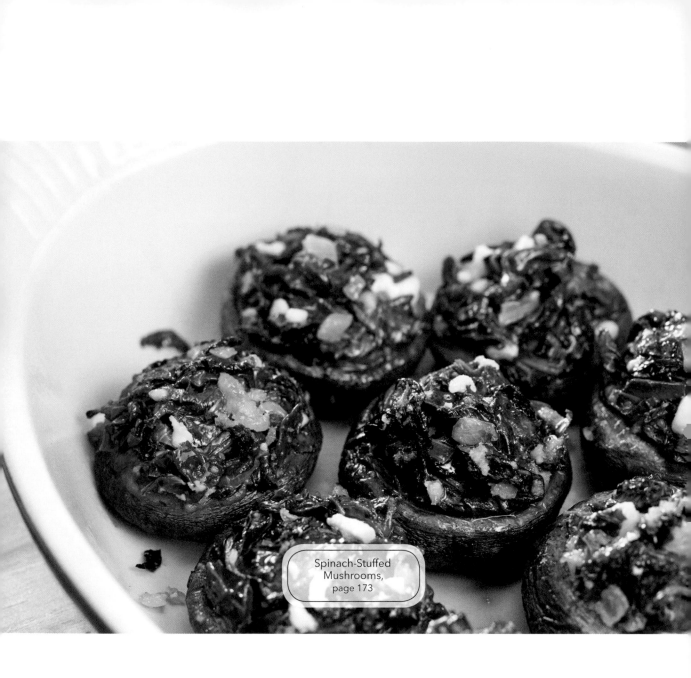

Spinach-Stuffed
Mushrooms,
page 173

SPINACH-STUFFED MUSHROOMS

SERVES 8 (serving size: 2 stuffed mushrooms)

Tender, juicy mushrooms filled with spinach and creamy tart cheese—unprocessing your diet just got more delicious. These stuffed mushrooms make an elegant presentation that's sure to impress!

Ingredients:

- 1 tablespoon grass-fed butter
- ¼ cup onion chopped
- 6 cups fresh baby spinach
- ¼ teaspoon freshly grated nutmeg
- 1 tablespoon almond flour
- ⅓ cup crumbled feta cheese
- ¼ teaspoon Himalayan salt
- ¼ teaspoon fresh ground black pepper
- 16 large button mushrooms, cleaned and stem cut off

Directions:

- ➤ Preheat oven to 375 degrees.
- ➤ In a medium skillet, melt butter over medium-high heat and sauté onions until translucent, about 2 minutes.
- ➤ Add spinach and cook until wilted, about 2 minutes.
- ➤ Remove from heat and add nutmeg, almond flour, and feta cheese. Salt and pepper to taste.
- ➤ Fill the mushroom cups with spinach and cheese, mix and place on a baking sheet. Bake for 15 minutes; mushrooms should be tender.

Calories: 89/Calories from fat: 60
Fat: 6.7g, Protein: 2.5g, Total carb: 5.4g, Fiber: 1.6g, Sugars: 1g, Sodium: 467mg, Vitamin A: 711mg, Vitamin C: 4.1mg, Calcium: 45mg, Iron: 0.9mg

Blackberry Goat Cheese
Meatless Sliders,
page 175

BLACKBERRY GOAT CHEESE MEATLESS SLIDERS

SERVES 8

Grilled eggplant gives a meaty feel to these Jump Start–style sliders that are both meatless and breadless. The surprise ingredients—creamy white cheese and sweet-tart blackberry sauce—add a flavor contrast and look pretty on the plate. If blackberries are unavailable, substitute raspberries.

Ingredients:

- 1 eggplant
- Himalayan salt and fresh ground black pepper
- 6 ounces goat cheese, crumbled Chevre log

Blackberry Dressing:

- ½ pint blackberries
- ¼ cup water
- 2 tablespoons balsamic vinegar
- 1 tablespoon extra virgin olive oil
- 1 teaspoon agave nectar (optional)
- 1 teaspoon fresh thyme, chopped
- ¼ teaspoon Himalayan salt
- ¼ teaspoon fresh ground pepper

Directions:

➤ Slice eggplant crosswise into 16 ¼-inch thick slices (save any leftovers for another use), lay it out on paper towel or platter and sprinkle with ½ teaspoon salt. Let it sit for about 10 minutes. This takes some of the bitterness out of the eggplant. Once the 10 minutes is up, pat dry.

➤ Preheat grill or grill pan to medium-high.

➤ In a blender, puree the blackberries with ¼ cup water until smooth.

➤ Press blackberries through a mesh strainer into a bowl; this should give you about ½ cup of juice.

➤ Whisk in the remaining ingredients.

➤ Lightly oil grill with olive oil cooking spray. Salt and pepper eggplant and place on the grill, cook until grill marks form and eggplant is tender, turning once halfway through grilling, about 4 to 6 minutes per side.

➤ When done, take eggplant off grill and top the eggplant while it is warm with the goat cheese, then drizzle the top with the blackberry dressing.

Calories: 137/Calories from fat: 85
Fat: 9.5g, Protein: 7.3g, Total carb: 6.8g, Fiber: 2.5g, Sugars: 4g, Sodium: 171mg, Vitamin A: 428mg, Vitamin C: 5mg, Calcium: 201mg, Iron: 0.7mg

RATATOUILLE

SERVES 8

This hearty summer stew is a bold and fresh-tasting take on a classic French dish. Serve alongside roasted chicken or another protein to complete your meal; vegetarians can add chickpeas, edamame, or a hard-boiled egg.

Ingredients:

¼ cup extra-virgin olive oil
1 medium onion, chopped
2 medium bell peppers, any
    color, cut into strips
1 medium zucchini, cubed
1 small eggplant, cubed
4 cloves garlic, minced
2 medium tomatoes, diced
1 bay leaf
1 teaspoon fresh basil
1 teaspoon fresh marjoram
½ teaspoon fresh oregano
3 tablespoons red cooking wine
½ cup tomato juice
2 tablespoons tomato paste
¾ teaspoon Himalayan salt
¼ teaspoon black pepper to taste

Directions:

➤ Heat oil in large high-sided skillet, add bay leaf, onion, and ½ teaspoon salt and saute over medium-high heat until slightly brown, about 10 minutes. Add garlic and cook until fragrant, about 30 seconds.

➤ Add eggplant, wine, tomato juice, basil, marjoram, and oregano, mix well, cover, and simmer for 10-15 minutes on low heat.

➤ When eggplant is tender, add the zucchini, peppers, tomatoes, tomato paste, and stir all ingredients until mixed in. Cover and simmer, stirring occasionally. Stew until all vegetables are tender, about 30 minutes. Season to taste with salt and pepper.

Calories: 130/Calories from fat: 68
Fat: 7.5g, Protein: 2.7g, Total carb: 13.7g, Fiber: 4g, Sugars: 8g, Sodium: 244mg, Vitamin A: 1865mg, Vitamin C: 74mg, Calcium: 34mg, Iron: 1.2mg

12
MAINS

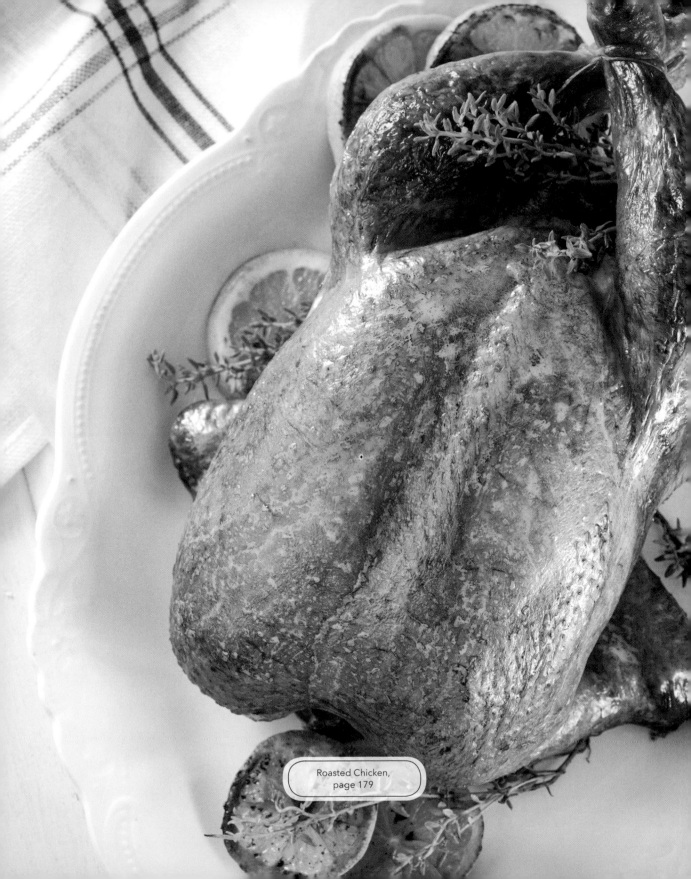

Roasted Chicken,
page 179

ROASTED CHICKEN

SERVES 4

There's nothing more comforting than roasted chicken. If you've never roasted your own chicken before, give it a try—I've got your back. The most important thing to do is to get yourself an instant-read thermometer, and when it hits 165 degrees, take your chicken out of the oven for the most moist, juicy results. You've got this!

Ingredients:

- 1 whole 3½ to 4 lbs organic roasting chicken, giblets (insides) removed
- 9 sprigs of fresh thyme
- Any additional fresh spices you might like to add (thyme, rosemary, basil, etc.)
- 2 teaspoons Himalayan salt
- ½ teaspoon fresh ground pepper
- 1 lemon, halved
- 4 cloves garlic, can use more if you like
- 2 tablespoons olive oil

Directions:

- ➤ Preheat oven to 450 degrees. Loosen the skin from the chicken breast and place ½ of the thyme, 1 teaspoon salt, and other seasoning of choice under the skin. Season the chicken inside and out with salt and pepper. Place the other half of the thyme, salt, and seasonings in the chicken cavity along with the garlic and lemon. Tress the chicken to seal in the juices while cooking.
- ➤ Place the chicken on a medium-size roasting pan. Brush or drizzle on olive oil.
- ➤ Roast chicken until a meat thermometer inserted into the thickest part of the thigh not touching the bones, registers 165 degrees, about 45 minutes to 1 hour.
- ➤ Remove chicken from oven when done and cover loosely with foil. Let stand for 15 minutes.

Calories: 358/Calories from fat: 210
Fat: 23.4g, Protein: 33.7g, Total carb: 1.2g, Fiber: 0.1g, Sugars: 0g, Sodium: 861mg, Vitamin A: 201mg, Vitamin C: 1mg, Calcium: 25mg, Iron: 1.7mg

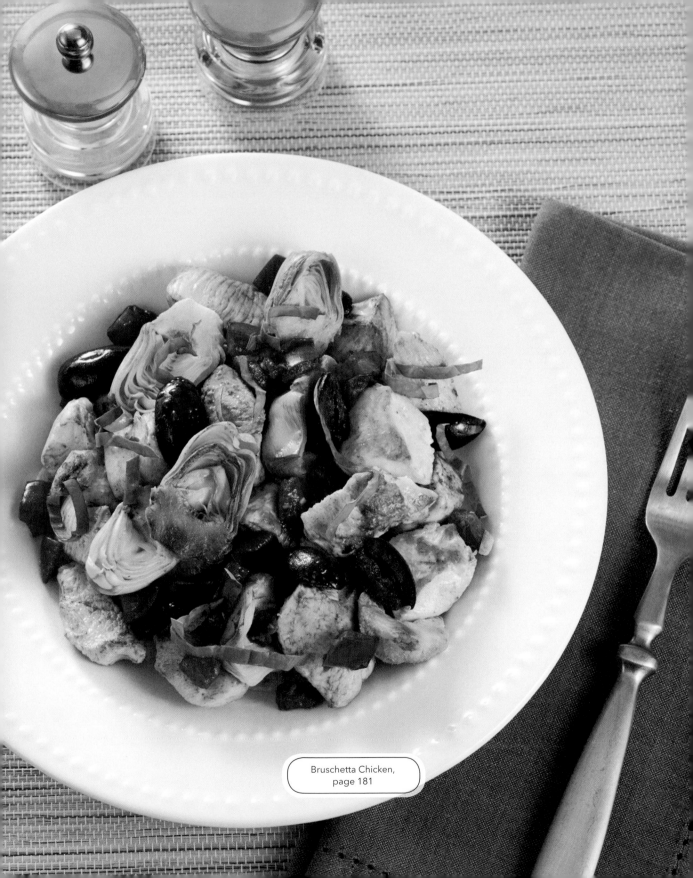

Bruschetta Chicken,
page 181

BRUSCHETTA CHICKEN

SERVES 4

The best part of bruschetta isn't the bread but what you put on top! So we've turned this Italian appetizer on its head by taking standard bruschetta toppings including tomatoes, garlic, and basil, and serving them over chicken for a tangy, salty, highly flavored full meal. If you're missing the bread, serve a slice of gluten-free toast alongside and count it as your carb for the meal.

Ingredients:

- 1½ lbs boneless-skinless chicken breasts, cut into ¾-inch pieces
- 6 ounces artichoke hearts from 1 13.75-ounce can in water, drained, quartered
- 6-8 basil leaves, thinly sliced, for garnish
- 2 cloves garlic, minced
- 1 large tomato diced
- 1 teaspoon Himalayan salt
- ½ teaspoon pepper
- 2 tablespoons olive oil
- 1 tablespoon balsamic vinegar

Directions:

➤ Season the chicken with garlic, salt, and pepper, heat oil in a skillet over medium-high heat, and cook the chicken pieces until golden brown, about 4–6 minutes. Remove them to a plate.

➤ Add diced tomato and cook until the juices are released, about 2–3 minutes. Then add the artichoke hearts and return the chicken back to the pan to warm through.

➤ Finish with the balsamic vinegar and cook until it's slightly caramelized and coats the chicken like a sauce.

➤ Garnish with fresh basil. Serve immediately.

Calories: 302/Calories from fat: 101
Fat: 11.4g, Protein: 38.9g, Total carb: 10.3g, Fiber: 1.9g, Sugars: 4g, Sodium: 849mg, Vitamin A: 828mg, Vitamin C: 29mg, Calcium: 26mg, Iron: 1.2mg

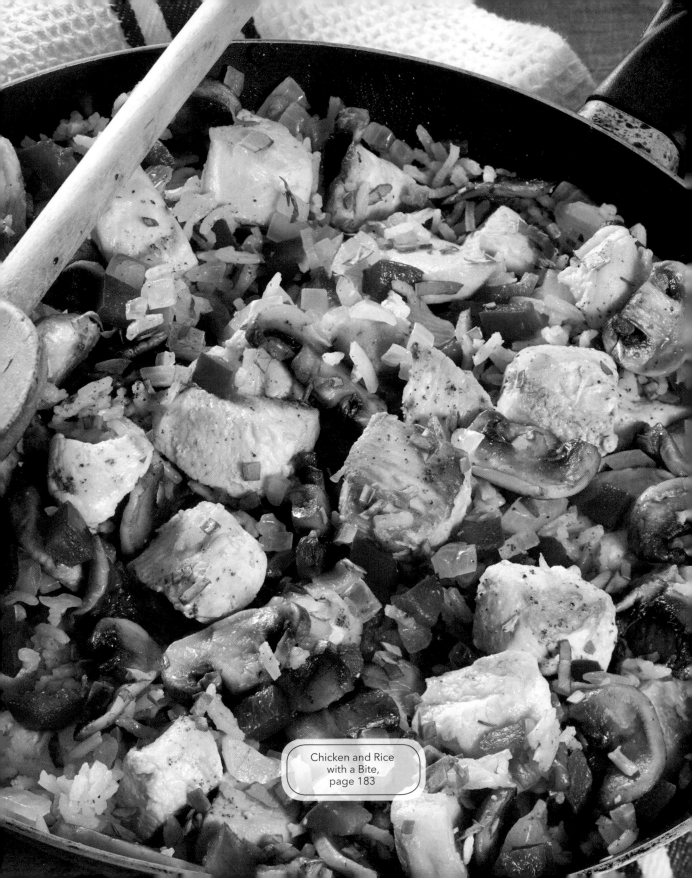

Chicken and Rice
with a Bite,
page 183

CHICKEN AND RICE WITH A BITE

SERVES 4

Perfect Natalie Jill–style comfort food with just the right kick of spice to keep you energized rather than stuffed and sleepy! Plenty of protein will keep you satisfied and feeling strong!

Ingredients:

- 2 tablespoons extra-virgin olive oil
- 1 lb boneless, skinless chicken breasts, cut into ¾" cubes
- ½ teaspoon Himalayan salt
- ½ teaspoon fresh ground pepper
- ½ chopped onion
- 1 cup sliced button mushrooms
- 1 red bell pepper
- 4 cloves garlic
- ½ cup long grain white rice
- 1½ cup homemade chicken broth
- 2 tablespoons coconut aminos
- ½ teaspoon cayenne pepper (if you prefer less spicy, drop down to ¼ teaspoon)
- 3 tablespoons fresh basil, chopped

Directions:

➤ In a large high-sided skillet with lid, heat oil on medium-high. Season chicken with ½ teaspoon salt and ½ teaspoon pepper and cook, stirring once or twice until lightly golden and almost cooked through, about 6 minutes.

➤ Add onions and cook until onions are just beginning to soften, about 2 minutes.

➤ Add mushrooms, peppers, and garlic and cook until peppers are crisp tender, about 3 minutes.

➤ Mix in rice, broth, coconut aminos, cayenne pepper, and bring to boil. Reduce heat, cover and, simmer until liquid is absorbed and rice is tender, about 25 minutes.

➤ Remove from heat, and let stand covered for an additional 10 minutes to let rice further absorb the liquid. Fluff with a fork, and mix in basil. Serve immediately.

Calories: 312/Calories from fat: 97
Fat: 11.1g, Protein: 26.8g, Total carb: 24.7g, Fiber: 1.6g, Sugars: 3g, Sodium: 378mg, Vitamin A: 1520mg, Vitamin C: 57mg, Calcium: 27mg, Iron: 1.7mg

Sun-Dried Tomato Chicken with Artichoke and Asparagus, page 185

SUN-DRIED TOMATO CHICKEN WITH ARTICHOKE AND ASPARAGUS

SERVES 5

This Mediterranean-inspired chicken dish is as simple as you'd like to make it: either start with a whole chicken (make it free-range and organic if at all possible) and roast it (page 179), use the leftover chicken from making chicken broth (page 147), or buy a ready-to-go roasted chicken.

Ingredients:

2 tablespoons olive oil
4 cloves garlic, minced
1 pound asparagus, trimmed and
    cut into 2-inch pieces
1 cup sun-dried tomatoes in oil,
    drained, julienned
1½ cups roasted chicken
1 cup artichoke hearts from
    1 14-ounce can packed in
    water, drained and quartered
½ cup fresh packed basil leaves
Himalayan salt and fresh ground
    pepper to taste

Directions:

➤ In a large skillet, heat oil over medium heat. Add garlic and cook until fragrant, about 30 seconds. Add asparagus and cook until crisp and tender, about 3 to 4 minutes.

➤ Add artichokes, sun-dried tomatoes, and chicken and cook, stirring occasionally until heated through, about 3 minutes. Fold in basil and salt and pepper to taste.

TIP: Save the asparagus trimmings to add to chicken broth (page 147) for added flavor.

Calories: 352/Calories from fat: 202
Fat: 22.6g, Protein: 24.5g, Total carb: 13.9g, Fiber: 4g, Sugars: 3g, Sodium: 880mg, Vitamin A: 1135mg, Vitamin C: 34mg, Calcium: 71mg, Iron: 2.7mg

CROCKPOT BALSAMIC CHICKEN AND VEGGIES

SERVES 4 (serving size: 2 thighs and about 1 cup sauce and vegetable mixture)

This dish is reason enough to go out and buy yourself a slow cooker! A satisfying meal of tangy, tender chicken and veggies will be your effortless reward.

Ingredients:

- 8 boneless, skinless chicken thighs
- 1 teaspoon Himalayan salt
- ½ teaspoon pepper to taste
- 2 cups carrots, sliced
- 2 cups celery, chopped
- ½ chopped onion
- 6 cloves garlic, minced
- 2 tablespoons basil leaves, thinly sliced, plus more for garnish
- ½ cup balsamic vinegar
- 1 tablespoon coconut nectar
- 3 tablespoons extra-virgin olive oil

Directions:

- ➤ Place chicken into the crockpot and season to taste with salt and pepper
- ➤ Place carrots, celery, onion, garlic, and basil on top of chicken. Do not stir.
- ➤ Pour in the balsamic vinegar, coconut nectar, and olive oil.
- ➤ Cover and cook on high for 4 hours until chicken is very tender. Serve immediately, garnished with basil leaves, if desired.

TIP: If you've thought of a slow cooker as "just one more appliance," think again. It can be a real time-saver and be an asset in an unprocessed lifestyle! A decent one can be had for under fifty dollars, and you'll love the smells wafting from the kitchen while your dinner (or breakfast!) cooks away.

Calories: 426/Calories from fat: 209
Fat: 23.7g, Protein: 38.6g, Total carb: 17.8g, Fiber: 3.6g, Sugars: 11g, Sodium: 624mg, Vitamin A: 4778mg, Vitamin C: 15mg, Calcium: 78mg, Iron: 2.6mg

CHICKEN-STUFFED PEPPERS

SERVES 4 (serving size: 1 stuffed pepper half)

A fun way to eat bell peppers, and a little cheese goes a long way to a satisfying stuffed pepper. This dish is great when you're looking for something a little special but don't have a whole lot of time to spend on making dinner. Stuffed peppers are perfect for serving when entertaining, and the whole family will love them!

Ingredients:

   3 red bell peppers
   1 tablespoon coconut oil
   ½ diced yellow onion
   4 cloves garlic, chopped
   ½ cup fresh diced tomatoes
   1 lb ground chicken white meat
   2 tablespoons feta cheese,
      crumbled
   1 tablespoon pine nuts
   ¼ cup chopped fresh basil
   ½ teaspoon Himalayan salt
   ¼ teaspoon fresh ground black
      pepper

TIP: Shop your local farmers' market in summer for yellow, chocolate brown, or orange-colored bell peppers to change things up.

Directions:

➤ Preheat oven to 375 degrees.

➤ Cut bell peppers in half, remove seeds. Lay them on a baking sheet skin side down; set aside.

➤ Heat coconut oil in a medium skillet over medium-high heat. Add onion and cook, stirring occasionally, until translucent, about 4 minutes. Add the garlic and tomatoes and let cook until warmed through, about 2 minutes. Add the ground chicken and cook until crumbled, about 6 minutes.

➤ Stir in basil and season with salt and pepper to taste.

➤ Spoon chicken mixture into each pepper half, place baking sheet in oven, and cook for 20–25 minutes.

➤ While peppers bake, cook pine nuts in a small skillet over medium heat, stirring constantly until lightly toasted, about 5 minutes; set aside.

➤ Top with feta (while warm) and sprinkle with toasted pine nuts.

Calories: 229/Calories from fat: 81.5
Fat: 9.2g, Protein: 26.6g, Total carb: 9.3g, Fiber: 2.5g, Sugars: 5g, Sodium: 380mg, Vitamin A: 2951mg, Vitamin C: 112mg, Calcium: 52mg, Iron: 1.2mg

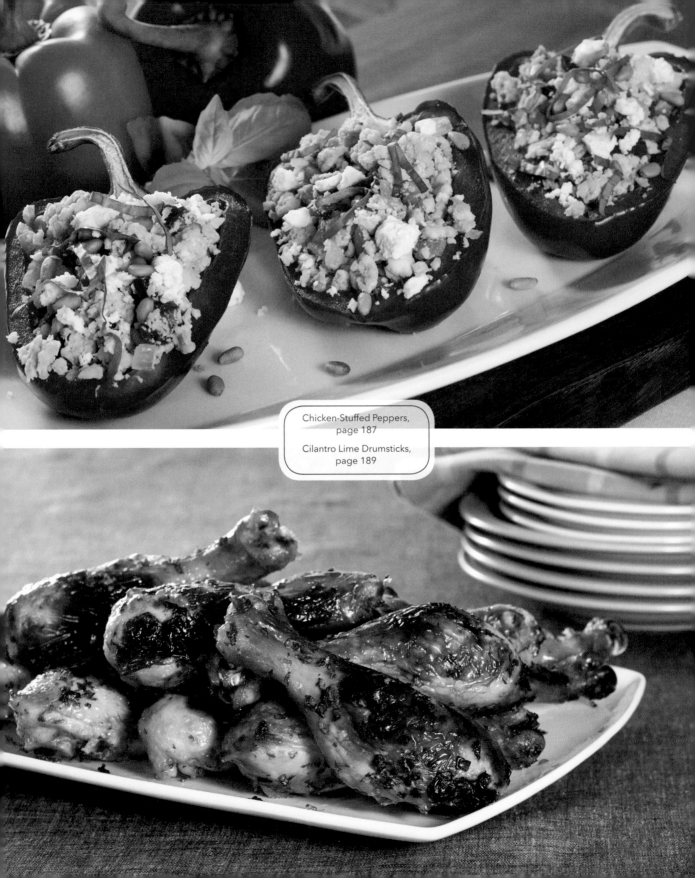

Chicken-Stuffed Peppers,
page 187

Cilantro Lime Drumsticks,
page 189

CILANTRO LIME DRUMSTICKS

SERVES 4 (serving size: 2 drumsticks)

Cilantro and lime are "free foods" on my Jump Start (see page 63), adding tons of flavor with next to no calories. Use free foods liberally to your taste buds' delight! The longer you marinate the chicken, the more the flavors will pop.

Ingredients:

2 teaspoons lime zest
½ cup fresh lime juice
¼ cup coconut nectar
½ cup chopped fresh cilantro
½ white onion, finely chopped
1 large jalapeño, seeded and
    minced
½ teaspoon Himalayan salt
½ teaspoon ground black pepper
8 drumsticks

Directions:

➤ Line a nonstick baking sheet with parchment paper or nonstick foil. Set aside.

➤ In a large ziptop bag, combine lime zest, lime juice, coconut nectar, cilantro, onion, and jalapeño, season with salt and pepper. Add chicken, seal bag, and marinate for 2 hours or overnight for more flavor.

➤ Heat oven to 425 degrees. Remove chicken from bag and place on prepared baking sheet. Discard any remaining marinade and bag. Roast turning once halfway through until chicken is cooked through and skin is golden, 40 to 45 minutes.

Calories: 330/Calories from fat: 160
Fat: 18g, Protein: 40g, Total carb: 0.7g, , Fiber: 0.1g, Sugars: 0g, Sodium: 230mg, Vitamin A: 103mg, Vitamin C: 2mg, Calcium: 27mg, Iron: 2.1mg

SWEET GINGER DRUMSTICKS

SERVES 3 (serving size: 2 drumsticks)

No worries about adding a touch of sweetness to your food, as long as your sweetener is an unprocessed one like agave or coconut nectar. So grab some drumsticks and invite a friend! Read more about unprocessing sugar from your diet on page 32. Add some steamed vegetables or a salad to make a complete meal.

Ingredients:

- 6 chicken drumsticks, skin peeled off
- ⅓ cup gluten-free Tamari (see page 192)
- 2 tablespoons coconut nectar
- 2 cloves garlic, minced
- 1 teaspoon fresh ginger, grated
- ⅛ to ¼ teaspoon crushed red pepper flakes

Directions:

➤ In a medium-size mixing bowl, whisk tamari, agave nectar, garlic, ginger, and crushed red pepper.

➤ Pour into a ziplock bag, add drumsticks, and shake to evenly coat drumsticks. Let marinate in refrigerator for minimum of an hour or overnight for better flavor.

➤ Preheat oven to 425 degrees. Line a baking sheet with parchment paper or nonstick foil.

➤ Place chicken legs on prepared baking sheet and bake, turning once, halfway through, until completely cooked and browned and caramelized in spots, 35 to 40 minutes.

Calories: 316/Calories from fat: 98
Fat: 10.9g, Protein: 49g, Total carb: 3.8g, Fiber: 0.2g, Sugars: 1g, Sodium: 1886mg, Vitamin A: 103mg, Vitamin C: 1mg, Calcium: 27mg, Iron: 3.2mg

SPICY CHICKEN STIR-FRY WITH GLUTEN-FREE SWEET SOY SAUCE

SERVES 2

Thai chili paste adds a great kick to this chicken and veggie stir-fry. Remember, you can swap in any protein from the protein swap-out list on page 59—try it with turkey or another lean meat to change it up. You can find palm sugar in Asian groceries; if unavailable, substitute unrefined dark brown sugar.

Ingredients:

- 2 tablespoons extra-virgin olive oil
- 2 garlic cloves, minced
- 2 tablespoons Thai roasted chili paste
- 8 ounces boneless-skinless chicken breast, sliced into thin pieces
- ¼ onion, cut into pieces
- 2 ounces green beans, tips removed and cut into 2-inch strips
- ½ small carrot, peeled and sliced
- ¼ green bell pepper, deseeded and thinly sliced
- ¼ red bell pepper or 1 red chili, deseeded and thinly sliced
- 1½ teaspoons sweet gluten-free soy sauce *see recipe below
- 1½ teaspoons coconut aminos

Directions:

➤ Heat a wok or large high-sided skillet on medium-high heat and add the oil. Add the garlic and stir-fry until aromatic, about 30 seconds, then add the Thai roasted chili paste. Add the chicken and quickly stir-fry, until the chicken is half cooked, about 2 to 3 minutes. Add the onion, green beans, carrot, green and red bell peppers, and stir to combine well with the chicken.

➤ Continue cooking, stirring constantly, until the vegetables are crisp tender and the chicken is cooked through, about 3 minutes. Add the sweet soy sauce and aminos, stir to blend well. If you want your chicken to be a little saucy, you can add two tablespoons of water. As soon as the chicken and all the ingredients are cooked through this dish is ready to serve.

continues

TIP: There are so many variations of this recipe: you can use cauliflower or broccoli instead of green beans, you can also add fresh corn, etc. The essence of the dish is in the sauce, not the vegetables used, so feel free to swap in your favorites.

Calories: 303/Calories from fat: 153
Fat: 17.7g, Protein: 26.2g, Total carb: 10.6g, Fiber: 2.7g, Sugars: 5g, Sodium: 554mg, Vitamin A: 2016mg, Vitamin C: 51mg, Calcium: 42mg, Iron: 1.1mg

SPICY CHICKEN STIR-FRY *continued*

GLUTEN-FREE SWEET SOY SAUCE
MAKES 10 TABLESPOONS (serving size: 1 tablespoon)

Ingredients:

¼ cup gluten-free Tamari
½ cup palm sugar

Directions:

➤ In small pot, add palm sugar and soy sauce.

➤ Boil the sauce over low to medium flame until it thickens, resembling maple syrup. If the mixture starts to boil vigorously and looks like it is going to overboil, move the pot away from the flame until the boiling has calmed down and continue to boil over low heat. You have to keep a watchful eye while the mixture is cooking to avoid over boiling. As the mixture cools down, it will further thicken.

Calories: 6/Calories from fat: 0
Fat: 0g, Protein: 0.8g, Total carb: 0.9g, Fiber: 0g, Sugars: 0g, Sodium: 376mg, Vitamin A: 0mg, Vitamin C: 0mg, Calcium: 3mg, Iron: 0.4mg

THAI CHICKEN WRAPS

DAY
4
LUNCH

SERVES 4 (serving size: 1 filled lettuce cup)

This absolutely delicious salad wrap makes for a full meal that won't leave you feeling hungry hours later. In true Thai style, this wrap is full of limey, spicy flavor. To keep it light, use lettuce leaves as your "wrappers."

Ingredients:

1 lb ground chicken
4 teaspoons coconut oil
4 cloves minced garlic
½ cup minced shallot
1 red bell pepper, sliced thin
2 serrano chiles, minced
2 teaspoons coconut aminos
1 cup fresh basil leaves
3 tablespoons fresh lime juice
¼ teaspoon fresh ground black
   pepper
4 lettuce leaves (butter lettuce or
   green leaf)
4 lime wedges
¼ cup chopped raw cashews
Pinch of salt

Directions:

➤ Heat large skillet to medium-high, add 2 teaspoons coconut oil, shallots, bell pepper, and garlic and cook, stirring occasionally until pepper is crisp tender, approximately 3-4 minutes. Remove mixture from pan.

➤ Add remaining 2 teaspoons coconut oil, and add chicken or (turkey) stirring to crumble and scrape up brown bits in the pan until browned, about 4 minutes. Drain juices.

➤ Add chiles and cook 1 minute, then add shallot mixture back to pan. Stir in coconut aminos and fresh ground pepper. Cook until heated through, about 1 to 2 minutes.

➤ Remove from heat and stir in basil and lime juice.

➤ Spoon into each lettuce leaf and serve with lime wedges.

TIP: For milder tastes, remove the seeds and membranes of the chiles, as that's where most of the heat is.

Calories: 276/Calories from fat: 150
Fat: 16.9g, Protein: 21.1g, Total carb: 12.5g, Fiber: 2.7g, Sugars: 4g, Sodium: 267mg, Vitamin A: 3657mg, Vitamin C: 66mg, Calcium: 55mg, Iron: 2.5mg

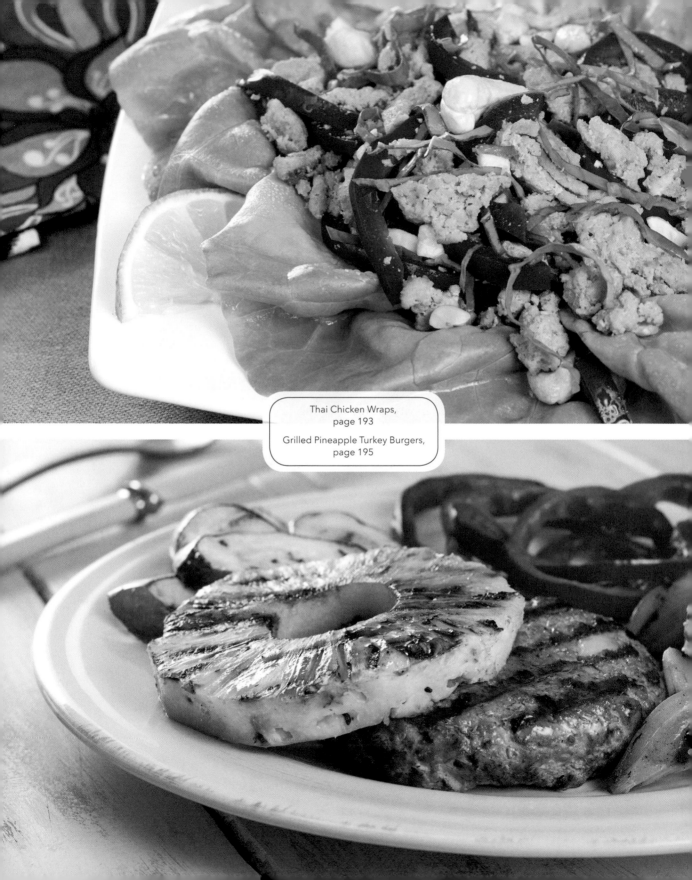

Thai Chicken Wraps,
page 193

Grilled Pineapple Turkey Burgers,
page 195

GRILLED PINEAPPLE TURKEY BURGERS

SERVES 4

Pineapple with your burger? You bet! It's a touch of Hawaii that I promise you'll turn to again and again. If you don't have access to an outdoor grill, you can grill both the burgers and pineapple inside on a grill pan set over medium-high heat. If you're missing the bun, nestle your burger into crisp lettuce leaves and have at it, fork and knife not required!

Ingredients:

- 1½ lbs ground white turkey meat
- 2 cloves garlic, minced
- 2 tablespoons fresh cilantro, chopped
- ½ yellow onion, chopped
- ½ teaspoon Himalayan salt
- ½ teaspoon fresh ground pepper
- 1 tablespoon olive oil
- 1 pineapple peeled, cored, and cut into 1" rings

Directions:

➤ Heat grill to medium-high.

➤ Place ground turkey, minced garlic, cilantro, onion, salt, and fresh ground pepper in a medium-size bowl. Mix with spoon or hands until all ingredients are well blended. Divide meat mixture into 4 even patties. Turn grill down to medium, lightly brush grill with olive oil and place patties on grates and grill, turning a few times until cooked through, about 7 minutes per side. Brush and oil grill if necessary. Grill pineapple rings 2–3 minutes per side and place 1 ring on top of each burger patty.

➤ Garnish with your favorite veggies.

TIP: Fresh pineapple is best here; if you use canned, make sure to buy fruit that has not been additionally sweetened or is packed in additive-laden syrup.

Calories: 290/Calories from fat: 39
Fat: 4.4g, Protein: 31.9g, Total carb: 32.3g, Fiber: 3.6g, Sugars: 23g, Sodium: 246mg, Vitamin A: 169mg, Vitamin C: 110mg, Calcium: 50mg, Iron: 2.3mg

TURKEY BACON CLUB WRAP

SERVES 4

A healthy lettuce wrap with the delicious taste of a BLT! For extra ease, grill the turkey ahead of time and have it handy in the fridge for on-the-spot sandwich making. Or substitute an equal amount of free-range sliced turkey from the deli.

Ingredients:

- 1 teaspoon Himalayan salt
- ½ teaspoon fresh ground pepper to taste
- 1 2-lb boneless skin-on turkey breast
- 2 teaspoons olive oil
- 4 green leaf lettuce leafs
- 4 slices of turkey bacon
- 1 vine tomato, halved and sliced into ¼ inch wedges
- 4 tablespoons goat cheese

Directions:

➤ Heat grill or grill pan on high until very hot.

➤ Salt and pepper the turkey breast. Drizzle the turkey with olive oil, place on grill, reduce grill to medium and cook covered, flipping once, halfway through cooking, until a thermometer inserted into the center registers 165 degrees, about 45 minutes to 1 hour. Transfer to a large plate and let rest until cool enough to handle, about 30 minutes.

➤ Meanwhile, place bacon slices in a medium skillet and cook over medium heat, turning occasionally, until crisp, about 12 to 15 minutes. Transfer to a paper towel-lined plate to drain and cool. Crumble and set aside.

➤ Remove skin from turkey breast and shred the turkey meat.

➤ Cut tomato slices in half.

➤ Lay out each green lettuce leaf, place shredded turkey evenly on each, then goat cheese, followed by tomato, then crumbled bacon. Be sure all ingredients are spread out on lettuce leaf, making it easier to roll. Roll each lettuce wrap up with all the ingredients inside, starting at one of the short ends, rolling all to the other.

Calories: 381/Calories from fat: 105
Fat: 11.8g, Protein: 62.4g, Total carb: 3g, Fiber: 0.9g, Sugars: 1g, Sodium: 1004mg, Vitamin A: 2223mg, Vitamin C: 8mg, Calcium: 58mg, Iron: 3.7mg

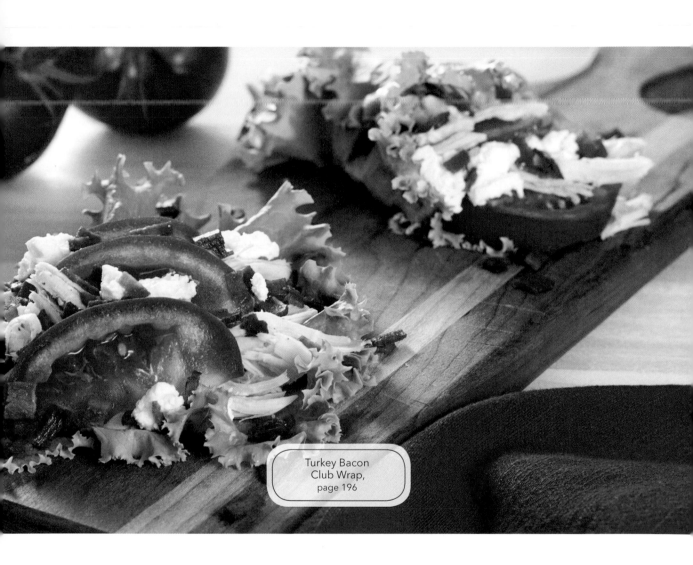

Turkey Bacon
Club Wrap,
page 196

AVOCADO AND SUN-DRIED TOMATO-STUFFED TURKEY BURGERS

SERVES 4

Sun-dried tomato and avocado add bold flavor and creamy texture to your burger. And the best part of the burger is that the flavor is stuffed *inside* it. So much so, you don't even need lettuce and tomato—but add them if you wish, because veggies are unlimited on the Jump Start!

Ingredients:

  2 medium avocados, ripe
  ½ cup sun-dried tomatoes, drained, julienned
  1 lemon, juiced
  2 lbs of ground white meat turkey
  1 teaspoon Himalayan salt
  ½ teaspoon pepper
  Oil for grill

Directions:

➤ Preheat grill or grill pan to medium heat.

➤ In a bowl, mash avocado and combine with sun-dried tomatoes and lemon juice. Set aside.

➤ Divide turkey into 8 equal balls. Use your hand to flatten each ball into a 4½"-diameter circle. Place approximately 3 heaping tablespoons of the avocado mixture on one patty, leaving a ½-inch border. Place the other patty on top, like a "sandwich," and pinch around the edges to seal the avocado mixture inside the two patties. Repeat until all ingredients are used. Season the outside of the burgers with salt and pepper to taste.

➤ Lightly oil grill with olive oil. Grill stuffed burgers, about 5 to 7 minutes per side, until cooked through (internal temp of 165 degrees). Let rest about 5 minutes for juices to redistribute before serving.

Calories: 443/Calories from fat: 179
Fat: 19.8g, Protein: 54.2g, Total carb: 13.6g, Fiber: 8.5g, Sugars: 1g, Sodium: 513mg, Vitamin A: 346mg, Vitamin C: 28mg, Calcium: 42mg, Iron: 3.6mg

NOODLE-FREE TURKEY VEGGIE LASAGNA

SERVES 9

Who needs noodles? You won't after eating this turkey eggplant take on the Italian classic, full of garlic, herbs, and just enough cheese to satisfy any lasagna lover. If you're dairy-free, just leave out the cheese—there's so much flavor, you won't miss it.

Ingredients:

- 1 tablespoon extra-virgin olive oil
- 1 small onion, diced
- 4 cloves garlic, minced
- 1 lb ground turkey or beef
- 1 28-ounce can crushed tomatoes (scant 2¾ cup)
- 1 6-ounce can tomato paste (scant ¾ cup)
- 1 teaspoon Himalayan salt
- ½ teaspoon pepper
- 1 large egg
- 16 ounces whole milk ricotta cheese
- ¾ cup grated parmesan cheese
- 1 tablespoon chopped fresh flat leaf parsley
- 1 tablespoon chopped fresh basil
- 8 ounces mozzarella cheese, grated
- 1 lb fresh spinach
- 1 large eggplant sliced vertically into ¼" thick slices

Directions:

➤ Preheat oven to 400 degrees.

➤ Sprinkle each eggplant slice with salt on both sides and let it sit until you are ready to start layering the lasagna. Pat each one dry before placing it in the baking dish.

➤ Heat oil in a large high-sided skillet over medium heat, add onion, and cook until slightly translucent, about 3 minutes. Add garlic and cook until fragrant, about 30 seconds. Add ground turkey (or beef) and cook, stirring occasionally, until cooked through and crumbled, about 8 minutes.

➤ Once turkey is fully cooked, add tomatoes, tomato paste, ½ teaspoon salt, and ½ teaspoon pepper. Reduce heat to medium-low, and simmer, stirring occasionally until thickened slightly, for 20 minutes.

➤ While the sauce is simmering, beat the egg in a medium bowl. Stir in ricotta cheese, ½ cup parmesan cheese, parsley, basil, salt, and pepper and set aside.

continues

Calories: 404/Calories from fat: 212
Fat: 23.5g, Protein: 30.5g, Total carb: 24.1g, Fiber: 6.9g, Sugars: 9g, Sodium: 916mg, Vitamin A: 2812mg, Vitamin C: 23mg, Calcium: 525mg, Iron: 4.5mg

NOODLE-FREE TURKEY VEGGIE LASAGNA *continued*

➤ In a separate, large high-sided skillet, cook spinach in batches over medium heat until wilted, about 15 minutes.

➤ Spread ⅓ meat sauce into bottom of a 9x13-inch baking dish. Lay down eggplant slices (or whatever you are replacing the pasta with). Sprinkle on ⅓ of the mozzarella cheese, ½ of the ricotta cheese mixture and ½ half of the spinach. Repeat the same layering process starting with the ⅓ meat sauce. After the spinach layer is finished top with the last ⅓ meat sauce sprinkle with the remaining mozzarella cheese and parmesan cheese.

➤ Cover with parchment paper oil side down and place foil on top.

➤ Place on a baking sheet to catch any drips. Cook for until eggplant is tender, about 45 minutes. Remove foil, return to oven and continue to cook until cheese is melted and bubbly, about 15 minutes. Let stand for 5 minutes before serving.

TIP: There are quite a few replacements for noodles. You can try zucchini, leeks, or even mashed sweet potatoes. You can also use the noodle layer to add more vegetables to your lasagna. You'll want to slice the eggplant and zucchini thin to get more of a noodle layer; otherwise, just add in whatever vegetables you choose. The sweet potatoes add a whole new twist of flavor. Of course, any changes will affect the nutritional profile somewhat.

HEARTY TURKEY AND VEGGIE STEW

SERVES 8

This hearty stew is a bit like turkey chili but without the beans and absolutely brimming with veggies. Turn off your electronic devices, pull up a bowl, and savor every last mouthful. Mindful eating makes your meals so much more satisfying; read more about the concept on page 69.

Ingredients:

- 1 tablespoon olive oil
- 2 lbs ground white meat turkey
- ½ teaspoon Himalayan salt
- 1 tablespoon butter, grass-fed
- 1 onion, chopped
- 2 stalks celery, chopped
- 1 red pepper, chopped
- 1 green pepper, chopped
- 2 carrots, chopped
- 2 cloves garlic, chopped
- 2 zucchini, chopped
- ½ teaspoon cumin
- 1 tablespoon chili powder
- ½ teaspoon red chili flakes
- 4 cups water or homemade chicken broth
- 2 cups tomatoes, pureed
- 1 cup corn kernels

Directions:

- ➤ Chop all vegetables and set aside. Keep the zucchini separate because that will be added last.
- ➤ Heat the olive oil in a large soup pot on medium-high, add turkey, season with ½ teaspoon salt, and cook until no longer pink and crumbled, about 10 minutes.
- ➤ Add the butter, onion, celery, peppers, carrots, and garlic, sauté for approximately 5 minutes until onion begins to soften. Then put in your seasonings, cumin, chili powder, chili flakes and salt, stir, and cook a few more minutes.
- ➤ Put in water or broth and pureed tomatoes, bring to a boil (about 4 minutes), cover and simmer until vegetables are very tender for 30 minutes.
- ➤ Then add in the zucchini and corn, mix in and simmer for an additional 15 minutes.
- ➤ Taste and add more cumin, chili powder, or red pepper flakes, if desired.

Calories: 239/Calories from fat: 54
Fat: 6g, Protein: 33.4g, Total carb: 16.2g, Fiber: 3.9g, Sugars: 8g, Sodium: 363mg, Vitamin A: 2804mg, Vitamin C: 65mg, Calcium: 39mg, Iron: 2.3mg

PESTO AND SUN-DRIED TOMATO TURKEY MEATLOAF

SERVES 8

Not a meatloaf fan? You will be after eating this. The secret? Pesto and sun-dried tomatoes add flavor; combined with the veggies, it's a moist, delicious meatloaf to remember.

Ingredients:

1 cup packed fresh basil
1 cup packed fresh spinach
¼ cup pine nuts
3 garlic cloves
½ cup plus 1 tablespoon olive oil
½ teaspoon salt
½ teaspoon pepper
½ cup sun-dried tomatoes, julienne-sliced and drained
1 large zucchini, shredded
1 large carrots, shredded
¼ cup button or crimini mushrooms, chopped
2 lbs of ground white meat turkey
1 large egg, whisked
1 onion, chopped
¼ cup tomato paste

Directions:

➤ Preheat oven to 375.

➤ In a high-speed blender or Vitamix, combine basil, spinach, pine nuts, garlic, olive oil, and salt and pepper. Blend on high until smooth to make a pesto sauce.

➤ In a large skillet over medium heat, add in 1 tablespoon olive oil; once olive oil heats, add the onion; once onion cooks to translucent (about 4 minutes), add zucchini, carrots, and mushrooms and sauté for 3-4 minutes or until the zucchini and carrots begins to soften.

➤ Transfer the cooked vegetables to a large bowl and let cool slightly, about 5 minutes. Combine the onion, carrot, zucchini, mushroom mixture with the ground turkey, egg, pesto, and sun-dried tomatoes.

➤ Pat the mixture into your loaf pan (5x9 inch) and smooth the top; bake for 1 hour.

➤ After the meatloaf has cooked for 1 hour, remove it from the oven and drain some of the fat out of the loaf pan if needed. Then brush the top of the meatloaf with the tomato paste and place back in the oven for about 15 minutes or until the top looks browned and caramelized.

➤ Drain some more fat out, if needed. Allow to rest for 10 minutes and serve.

Calories: 355/Calories from fat: 182
Fat: 20.5g, Protein: 33.8g, Total carb: 9.1g, Fiber: 2.4g, Sugars: 3.8g, Sodium: 223mg, Vitamin A: 1691mg, Vitamin C: 19mg, Calcium: 44mg, Iron: 2.9mg

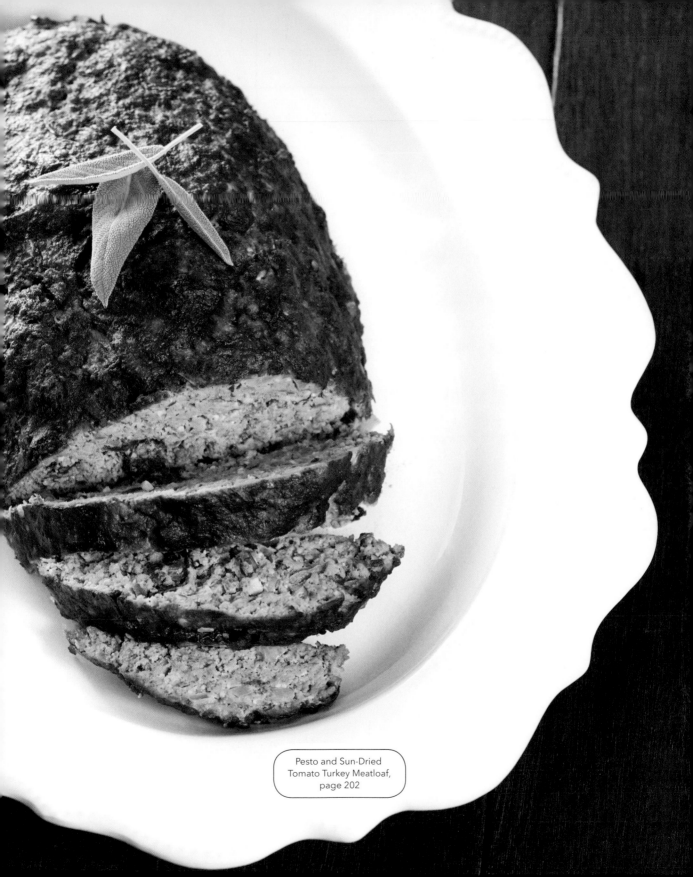

Pesto and Sun-Dried
Tomato Turkey Meatloaf,
page 202

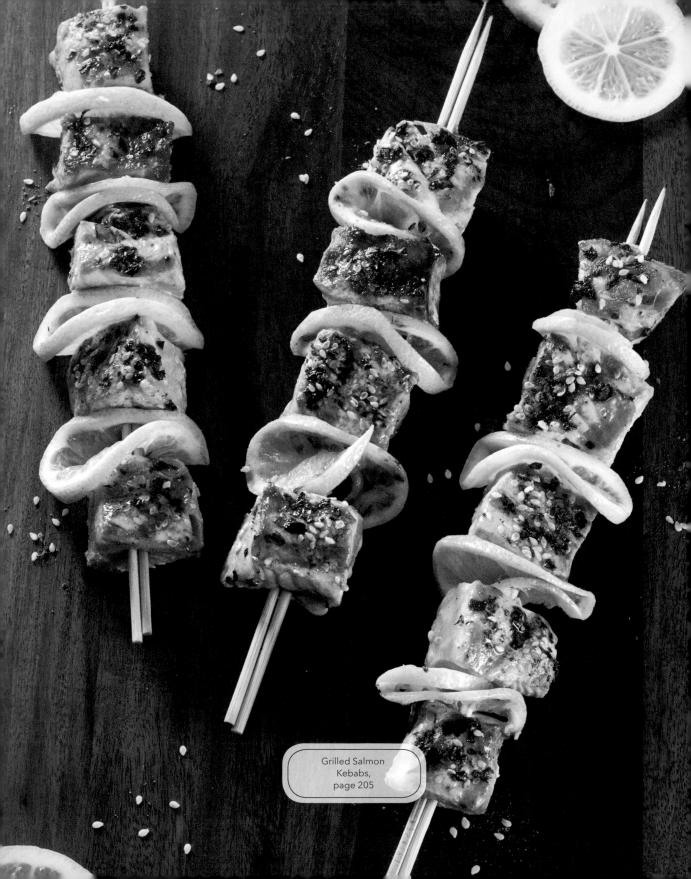

Grilled Salmon
Kebabs,
page 205

GRILLED SALMON KEBABS

SERVING SIZE: 4

A spice mixture featuring fresh oregano, cumin, and hot red pepper flakes flavors the salmon, with sesame seeds adding a little crunch. Feel free to substitute any other firm-fleshed fish for the salmon if you like.

Ingredients:

- 2 tablespoons chopped fresh oregano
- 2 teaspoons raw sesame seeds
- 1 teaspoon ground cumin
- ¼ teaspoon crushed red pepper flakes
- 1½ lbs boneless skinless wild salmon fillet, cut into 1-inch pieces
- 2 lemons, very thinly sliced into rounds
- 1 teaspoon pink Himalayan salt
- 16 bamboo skewers soaked in water for1 hour
- 1 teaspoon olive oil

Directions:

- ➤ Heat the grill or grill pan to medium-high heat.
- ➤ Mix oregano, sesame seeds, cumin, and red pepper flakes in a small bowl to combine; set spice mixture aside.
- ➤ Beginning and ending with the salmon, thread salmon and folded lemon slices onto 8 pairs of parallel skewers to make 8 kebabs total.
- ➤ Spray the fish lightly with oil, and season with kosher salt and the reserved spice mixture.
- ➤ Lightly dust the grill with oil. Place fish on grill and cook, turning occasionally, until fish is opaque throughout, about 8 to 10 minutes total.

TIP: Make sure to cut your salmon into equal-size pieces so it cooks evenly on the skewers.

Servings: 4 • Size: 2 kebabs
Calories: 242/Calories from fat: 129
Fat: 14.3g, Protein: 26.1g, Total carb: 0.6g, Fiber: 0.2g, Sugars: 0g, Sodium: 442mg, Vitamin A: 670mg, Vitamin C: 7mg, Calcium: 48mg, Iron: 0.6mg

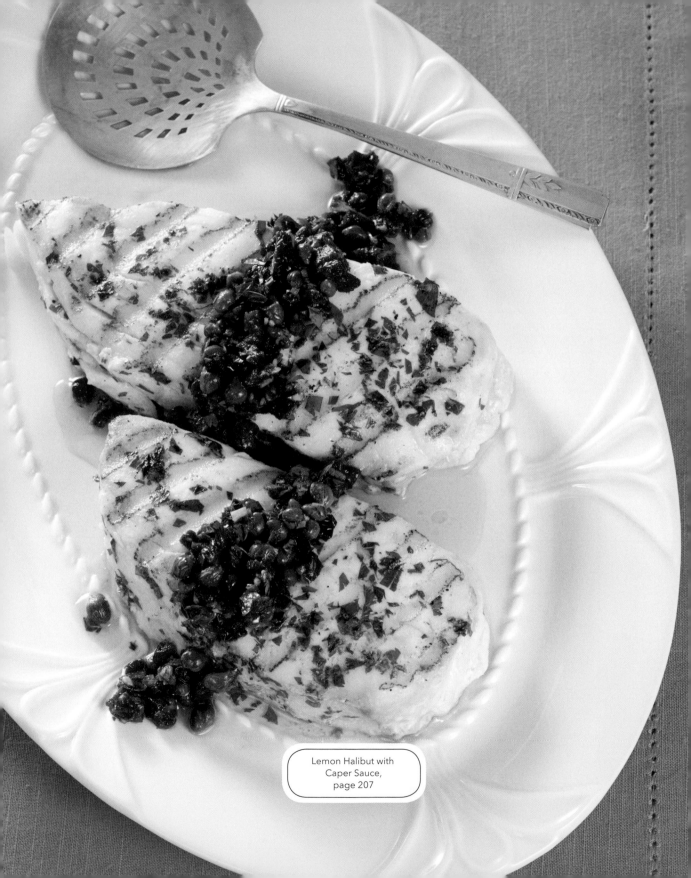

Lemon Halibut with
Caper Sauce,
page 207

LEMON HALIBUT WITH CAPER SAUCE

SERVINGS 4 (Serving Size: 1 fillet and about 2 tablespoons sauce)

Briefly marinating your fish infuses it with lemon-herb flavor, and a caper and sun-dried tomato sauce finishes the dish with a Mediterranean touch. A most delicious way of getting in your omega-3s! Read more about the importance of getting your omega-3 fatty acids from fish sources on page 47.

Ingredients:

For the Paste
2 tablespoons extra virgin olive oil
1 tablespoon finely chopped fresh Italian parsley
1 teaspoon grated lemon zest
¼ teaspoon Himalayan salt
¼ teaspoon ground black pepper
4 skinless halibut fillets (about 1¼ inch thick)

For the Sauce
2 tablespoons extra virgin olive oil
2 tablespoons fresh lemon juice
2 tablespoons finely chopped sun-dried tomatoes
2 tablespoons capers
1 tablespoon finely chopped fresh parsley
¼ teaspoon crushed red pepper flakes
¼ teaspoon Himalayan salt

Directions:

➤ In a small bowl, whisk together the paste ingredients.

➤ Rub the halibut on all sides with the paste. Cover with plastic wrap and refrigerate and marinate, about 15 minutes.

➤ In another bowl, whisk together the sauce ingredients. Set aside at room temperature.

➤ Heat a grill or grill pan to medium-high. Grill the fillets until the fish is just opaque at the center and slightly firm to the touch, 8-10 minutes to time turning once halfway through. Remove from the grill and serve warm with the sauce spooned on top.

Calories: 310/Calories from fat: 147
Fat: 16.7g, Protein: 36.7g, Total carb: 2.1g, Fiber: 0.4g, Sugars: 1g, Sodium: 482mg, Vitamin A: 411mg, Vitamin C: 6mg, Calcium: 26mg, Iron: 0.7mg

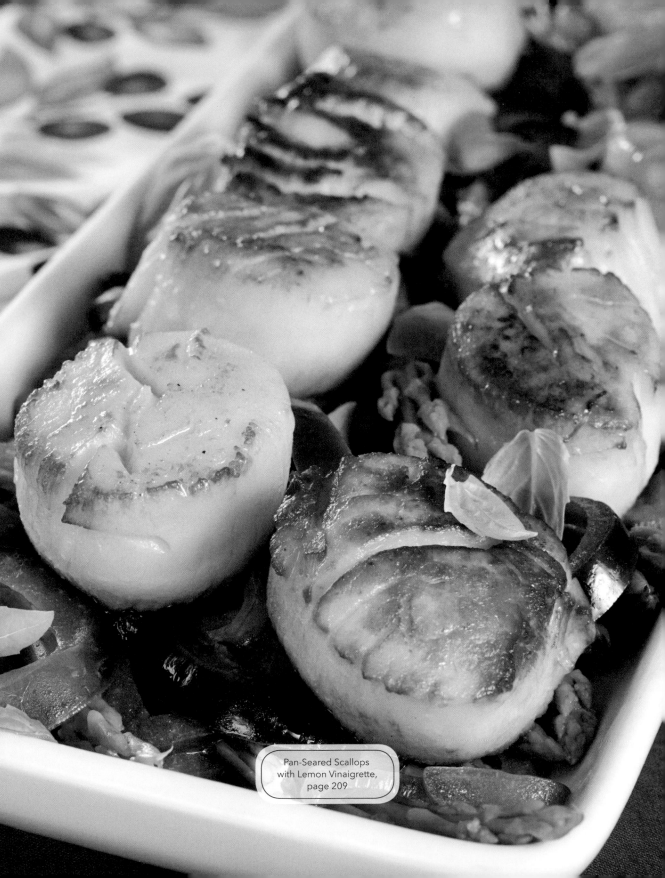

Pan-Seared Scallops
with Lemon Vinaigrette,
page 209

PAN-SEARED SCALLOPS WITH LEMON VINAIGRETTE

SERVES 4

Buttery, sweet, and rich—scallops are a special treat that you can make any night, and they go from pan to plate in just a matter of minutes. Keeping your scallops simple, with few added embellishments, lets their natural flavor shine through.

Ingredients:

- 12 ounces fresh dry sea scallops
- 2 lemons
- 3 tablespoons extra-virgin olive oil
- 1 lb asparagus spears, trimmed and cut into 2-inch pieces
- 1 medium red onion, cut into wedges
- ½ teaspoon Himalayan salt
- ¼ teaspoon black pepper
- 2-3 basil sprigs with stem
- 2 tablespoons fresh basil leaves cut into strips (¼ ounce)

TIP: To cook your scallops just right: place them on the pan in a circular fashion and turn them in the same order you put them into the pan. You'll know they're done when they have a slight spring to them when touched, a nicely browned crust, and a mouth-wateringly tender center.

Directions:

➤ Rinse scallops and pat dry, set aside.

➤ Use a vegetable peeler to peel 1 lemon into long strips. Be careful not to peel off any of the bitter white pith.

➤ Heat 1 tablespoon olive oil in skillet over medium heat. Add the onion and cook until beginning to soften, about 4 minutes. Add the asparagus and cook until crisp tender, about 4 minutes. Season to taste with salt and pepper. Transfer to a serving platter and keep warm.

➤ Combine the lemon peel, basil sprigs, and remaining 2 tablespoons olive oil in the skillet. Cook for 1 minute, until heated through. Remove the lemon peel and basil sprigs with slotted spoon, leaving the oil in the skillet and discard.

➤ Pat scallops dry and season to taste with salt and pepper. Cook the scallops in the hot oil, flipping once, halfway through cooking until caramelized and opaque, about 3 minutes per side. Stir in the reserved lemon juice.

➤ Place the scallops over the asparagus mixture. Cut the remaining lemon into wedges. Garnish the scallops with the lemon wedges and basil if desired.

Calories: 251/Calories from fat: 103
Fat: 11.4g, Protein: 25.3g, Total carb: 12.7g, Fiber: 2.7g, Sugars: 4g, Sodium: 453mg, Vitamin A: 621mg, Vitamin C: 20mg, Calcium: 63mg, Iron: 2.6mg

GARLIC SHRIMP

SERVES 3

Lemon, garlic, and parsley flavor your shrimp Italian-style. If you buy your shrimp pre-peeled, this dish can be put together in five minutes. Even the busiest of us have five minutes for dinner! Shrimp are packed with protein, vitamins, and minerals and have a negligible amount of carbs, making them a perfect Jump Start protein companion.

Ingredients:

- 1 lb peeled and deveined shrimp, tails removed
- ¼ cup organic butter
- 2 cloves garlic
- 1 cup chopped parsley
- Himalayan salt and pepper to taste
- 1 tablespoon fresh lemon juice

Directions:

➤ Melt butter in medium skillet over medium heat; once butter is melted, add garlic and cook until fragrant, about 30 seconds. Put shrimp in and cook, stirring occasionally, until pink, curled, and opaque, about 4 minutes. Remove from heat and add parsley, salt and pepper. Stir to combine. Add lemon juice over top when serving, or squeeze on top in skillet as part of the sauce.

Calories: 253/Calories from fat: 147
Fat: 16.4g, Protein: 21.4g, Total carb: 3.8g, Fiber: 0.7g, Sugars: 0g, Sodium: 1121mg, Vitamin A: 2382mg, Vitamin C: 30mg, Calcium: 114mg, Iron: 1.6mg

SPANISH-STYLE SHRIMP

SERVES 3

Shrimp with garlic—what's not to love? Always a winning duo! This light but filling dish is the answer to dinner when time is short but you're not willing to skimp in the flavor department. And all that garlic will nourish your heart and stave away colds and flu!

Ingredients:

- 1 tablespoon extra-virgin olive oil
- ⅛ teaspoon ground red pepper
- 6 cloves of garlic, minced
- 1 bay leaf
- 1 lb peeled and deveined shrimp, tails removed
- ¼ teaspoon Himalayan salt
- 2 tablespoons chopped fresh parsley
- 1 lemon, cut in half

Directions:

➤ Heat oil in a medium nonstick skillet (cast iron skillet would work as well), over medium heat. Add pepper, garlic, and bay leaf; cook, stirring constantly until fragrant, about 2 minutes. Increase heat to medium-high, add shrimp and sauté until pink or opaque flesh, about 4 minutes. Remove from heat, discard bay leaf, sprinkle with salt and parsley, and serve with lemon wedges.

Calories: 184/Calories from fat: 59
Fat: 6.6g, Protein: 25.3g, Total carb: 4.7g, Fiber: 0.5g, Sugars: 0g, Sodium: 1156mg, Vitamin A: 574mg, Vitamin C: 10mg, Calcium: 115mg, Iron: 0.7mg

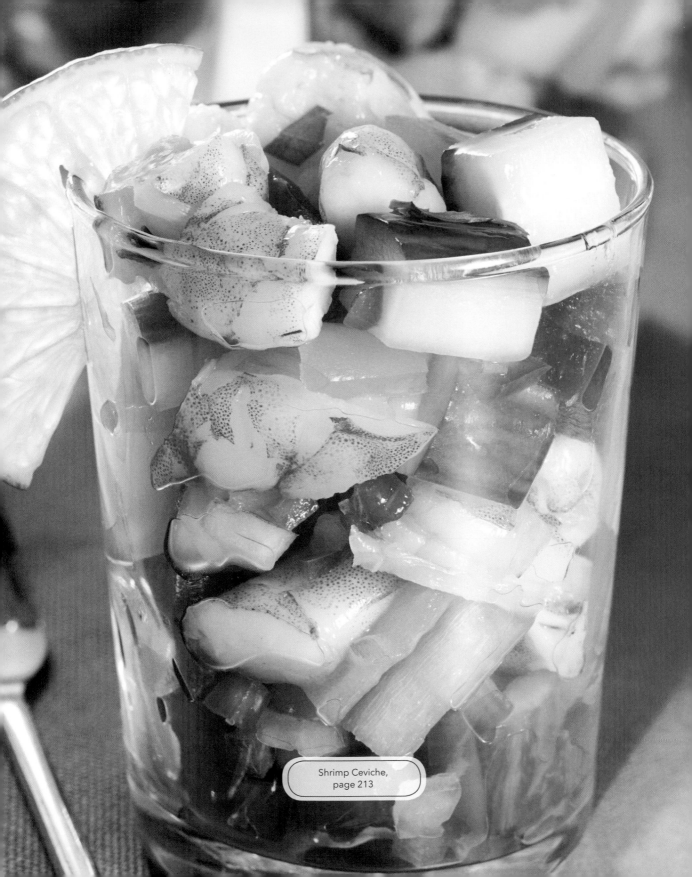

Shrimp Ceviche,
page 213

SHRIMP CEVICHE

DAY
6
LUNCH

SERVES 4

This recipe is perfect for first-time ceviche makers, as it starts with cooked shrimp, removing the intimidation factor from this typically raw fish dish. We marinate it in lemon and lime and add a hint of heat for a flavorful and refreshing ceviche.

Ingredients:

1 lb cooked shrimp, peeled, deveined, and tails removed
½ chopped red bell pepper
½ chopped yellow bell pepper
½ jalapeño, seeded and minced
½ cup chopped cucumber, skin on
2 tablespoons chopped fresh cilantro
1 tablespoon chopped shallot
Juice of 1 lime
Juice of 1 lemon
2 tablespoons extra-virgin olive oil

Directions:

➤ Cut each cooked shrimp into quarters and place in medium-size bowl.

➤ Add red and yellow bell peppers, jalapeño, cucumber, cilantro, shallot, juice of lime, juice of lemon, and olive oil. Mix well.

➤ Cover and refrigerate for a minimum of 30 minutes for flavor to come through before serving.

TIP: If your fish counter has wild American shrimp, choose them for their sweet, delicious flavor. Eating wild is cleaner too, as farm-raised shrimp have been found to contain higher levels of chemicals than wild shrimp.

Calories: 197/Calories from fat: 68
Fat: 7.5g, Protein: 27.9g, Total carb: 5.4g, Fiber: 1.1g, Sugars: 3g, Sodium: 129mg, Vitamin A: 1238mg, Vitamin C: 60mg, Calcium: 88mg, Iron: 0.8mg

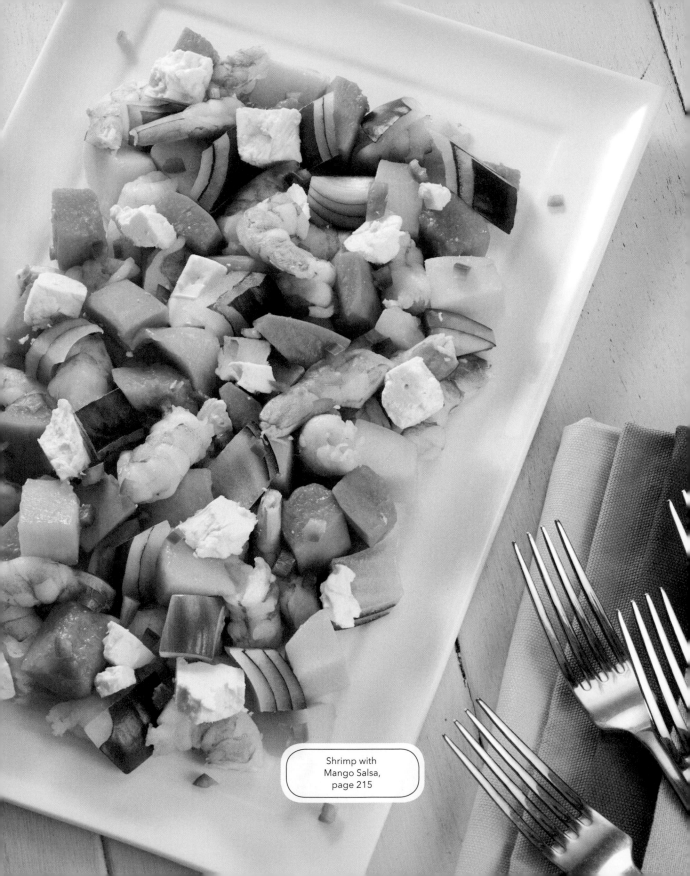

Shrimp with
Mango Salsa,
page 215

SHRIMP WITH MANGO SALSA

DAY
5
LUNCH

SERVES 4 (serving size: 2½ cups)

Shrimp is accented with salty cheese and a light, tropical salsa with bright, fresh flavors. If you're planning ahead, combine all the ingredients except the cheese, cover, and refrigerate for a few hours, and you'll be rewarded with flavors that really pop. Remove from the refrigerator a few minutes before serving to take off the chill, toss in the cheese, and serve.

Ingredients:

    1 mango ripe, diced cut into ¾"
    1 papaya ripe, diced cut into ¾"
    ½ bunch fresh cilantro, chopped
    1 jalapeño, finely chopped
    1 medium purple onion, cut into
        ¾" chop
    5 ounces crumbled feta cheese
    1 lb (31–40-count) cooked shrimp,
        peeled and deveined, cut into
        ¾" pieces

Directions:

➤ In a large bowl, combine mango, papaya, cilantro, jalapeño, and purple onion.

➤ Add the shrimp and feta cheese to the bowl and toss gently to combine.

TIP: Buy precooked shrimp on those hot summer days when you'd rather not turn on the stove. It will save you prep time, too.

Calories: 318/Calories from fat: 77
Fat: 8.5g, Protein: 33.4g, Total carb: 28.9g, Fiber: 3.4g, Sugars: 12g, Sodium: 533mg, Vitamin A: 2745mg, Vitamin C: 70mg, Calcium: 287mg, Iron: 1.2mg

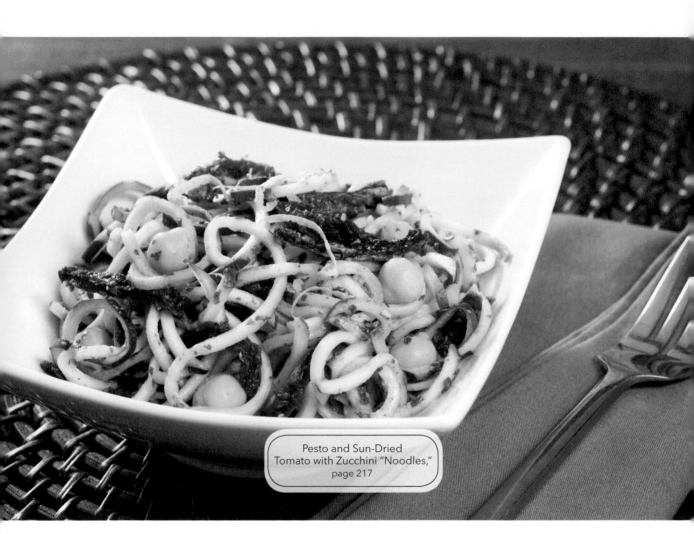

Pesto and Sun-Dried Tomato with Zucchini "Noodles," page 217

SPIRALIZE IT!

WHEN you remove wheat from your diet, you don't need to give up noodles. I've got a new type of noodle for you! It looks like a noodle, is full of flavor, but is gluten-free and practically carb-free. Introducing the spiralizer, a handy, relatively inexpensive little device sold in most kitchen stores, that cranks out spaghetti or ribbony noodle shapes from zucchini, carrots, turnips, and other vegetables. Spiralized noodles can be served either cooked or raw. If you don't want to invest in a spiralizer, a julienne peeler is a simple option.

PESTO AND SUN-DRIED TOMATO WITH ZUCCHINI "NOODLES"

SERVES 4

A Jump Start alternative to a carb-loaded pasta meal: a mega-green pesto containing both basil and spinach pumps it up with flavor. You've got two options—one with shrimp for seafood lovers and one with chickpeas for vegetarians and vegans.

Ingredients:

- ½ cup packed fresh basil, plus more for topping
- ½ cup packed fresh spinach
- 3 tablespoons toasted pine nuts
- 3 tablespoons olive oil
- 3 garlic cloves, chopped
- 1 teaspoon Himalayan salt
- ½ teaspoon pepper to taste
- 1 pound of raw shrimp, peeled, deveined, and tails removed*
- 4 large zucchini, spiralized or thinly sliced
- ½ cup sun-dried tomatoes, julienne sliced and drained
- 1 teaspoon olive oil
- Zest of 1 lemon
- *You may substitute 1 cup rinsed and drained chickpeas for the shrimp for a meatless meal.

Directions:

➤ In a high-speed blender or Vitamix, combine basil, spinach, garlic, 2 tablespoons olive oil, and salt and pepper to make a pesto sauce; water may be added to aid in blending if needed.

➤ Dust a large high-sided skillet with olive oil and warm over medium-high heat. Add raw shrimp and cook until opaque and curled and just cooked through on both sides, about 2 minutes per side. Transfer to a plate to set aside.

➤ In the same skillet, over medium heat, add more cooking spray and the zucchini "noodles" and cook, tossing with tongs occasionally until the zucchini begins to soften, about 5 minutes.

➤ Add in the cooked shrimp (or chickpeas), sauté for 1 to 2 additional minutes to warm through, and remove from heat.

➤ Stir in the pesto sauce, sun-dried tomatoes, lemon zest, season to taste with salt and pepper, and toss to combine.

➤ Serve garnished with fresh basil and pine nuts. Serve immediately.

Shrimp Version: Serves 4

Calories: 295/Calories from fat: 150
Fat: 16.9g, Protein: 21g, Total carb: 18.9g, Fiber: 4.7g, Sugars: 10g, Sodium: 983mg, Vitamin A: 1558mg, Vitamin C: 68mg, Calcium: 147mg, Iron: 2.9mg

Chickpea Version: Serves 4

Calories: 305/Calories from fat: 157
Fat: 17.6g, Protein: 11.1g, Total carb: 31.4g, Fiber: 4.6g, Sugars: 11g, Sodium: 590mg, Vitamin A: 1180mg, Vitamin C: 70mg, Calcium: 111mg, Iron: 3.3mg

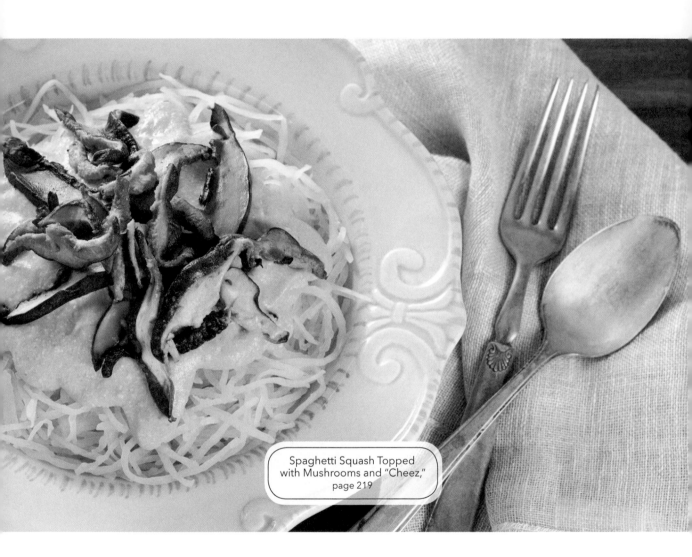

Spaghetti Squash Topped
with Mushrooms and "Cheez,"
page 219

SPAGHETTI SQUASH TOPPED WITH MUSHROOMS AND "CHEEZ"

SERVES 6

Impress vegans and meat-eaters alike with this wonderfully "cheezy" sauce made from nuts and seeds. Don't be surprised when you're asked for the recipe. Topped with "noodles" made from spaghetti squash, we've slashed the carbs and calories while upping both the fiber and the fun factor!

Ingredients:

- 1 large spaghetti squash
- 2 medium yukon gold potatoes, peeled and diced
- 1 medium carrot, peeled and diced
- ⅔ cup yellow onion, diced
- ⅓ cup coconut oil
- ⅓ cup raw cashews
- ⅓ cup raw macadamia nuts
- ¼ cup hemp seeds, hulled
- ¼ teaspoon dry mustard
- 2 tablespoons fresh lemon juice
- 2 cloves garlic
- 2 teaspoons Himalayan salt
- ½ teaspoon ground black pepper
- ¼ teaspoon cayenne pepper
- 2 cups shiitake mushrooms, stems removed, sliced
- 2 cups portobello mushrooms, stems removed and cut into quarters
- 1 tablespoon olive oil

Directions:

➤ Cut spaghetti squash in half lengthwise, remove seeds and inner portions of squash. Season with salt and pepper, place both halves face-down on a baking sheet. Roast for about 50 minutes at 375 degrees; the skin will soften and flesh will become translucent in color.

➤ While the squash is roasting, combine the potatoes, carrot, onion, and water in a saucepan over medium heat. Bring to a boil, about 12 minutes, reduce heat, cover and simmer for 10 minutes or until the vegetables are tender. Reserve 1 cup vegetable cooking liquid. Drain vegetables.

➤ Once the vegetables are done put them in a blender with the 1 cup of reserved liquid. Add oil, cashews, macadamia nuts, hemp seeds, salt, garlic, lemon juice, mustard, black pepper, and cayenne. Blend until completely smooth.

continues

Calories: 396/Calories from fat: 241
Fat: 27.4g, Protein: 7.9g, Total carb: 33.7g, Fiber: 5.7g, Sugars: 9g, Sodium: 560mg, Vitamin A: 1343mg, Vitamin C: 22mg, Calcium: 67mg, Iron: 2.9mg

SPAGHETTI SQUASH TOPPED WITH
MUSHROOMS AND "CHEEZ" *continued*

➤ Heat olive oil in a medium skillet on medium heat. Cook the mushrooms in the skillet with oil; they will start to release their own juices. Continue cooking until browned. About 5 minutes.

➤ When the spaghetti squash is done and cooled, pull the flesh from the inside with a fork and place in a bowl.

➤ Place the cooked spaghetti squash onto 4 serving plates, pour "cheez" on squash, and top with cooked mushrooms.

➤ Freeze leftovers for another time and cook fresh mushrooms.

VEGAN BURGERS

SERVES 6

Packed full of protein from chickpeas and edamame, these burgers are a far cry from the processed cardboard-tasting variety you get from the freezer section. Guaranteed to please vegans, vegetarians, and meat-eaters alike. Top with a dab of lime guacamole and you're all set!

Ingredients:

2 cups canned, unsalted chickpeas, rinsed and drained, separated
½ cup dried lentils, rinsed
½ cup cooked quinoa
¼ cup oat bran
¼ cup warm water mixed with 1½ tablespoons ground flax
2 cloves of garlic, minced
¼ cup red onion, chopped
½ red pepper, finely chopped
¼ cup walnuts, chopped
½ tablespoon ground cumin
¼ teaspoon cayenne
½ teaspoon Sriracha (or other hot sauce)
½ teaspoon Himalayan salt
⅛ teaspoon freshly ground black pepper
¼ cup lime guacamole (see page 157)
2 cups of thawed and shelled edamame

Directions:

➤ Preheat the oven to 375 degrees.

➤ Bring 4 cups of water to a boil over high heat, about 8 minutes. Do not add any salt.

➤ Add the lentils to the boiling water, let cook for 5 minutes, then reduce to a simmer until lentils are tender, 10-15 minutes. Drain the excess water and rinse the lentils until the water runs clear. Set aside.

➤ Combine the ground flax with the warm water and let sit for 10 minutes.

➤ Puree the lentils with 1 cup of the chickpeas. Pour into a large bowl and mix with the remaining 1 cup of chickpeas, quinoa, oat bran, garlic, red onion, red pepper, walnuts, flax seed water combination, and spices.

➤ Refrigerate the mixture for 1 hour (time will make it easier to form patties).

➤ To form the patties, grab a handful of the patty mixture and form it into a ball. It may be a bit sticky. Drop onto a parchment-lined sheet, and press down lightly with your fingers to flatten. Repeat with remaining mixture, to form a total of 4 patties. Bake until heated through, about 24 minutes. Gently transfer the burgers to 4 plates. Top each burger with 1 tablespoon of lime guacamole, and serve with ½ cup of edamame per person.

Totals include lime guacamole.
Calories: 314/Calories from fat: 96
Fat: 10.6g, Protein: 15.5g, Total carb: 42.2g, Fiber: 11.9g, Sugars: 3.5g, Sodium: 445mg, Vitamin A: 517mg, Vitamin C: 25mg, Calcium: 71mg, Iron: 3.7mg

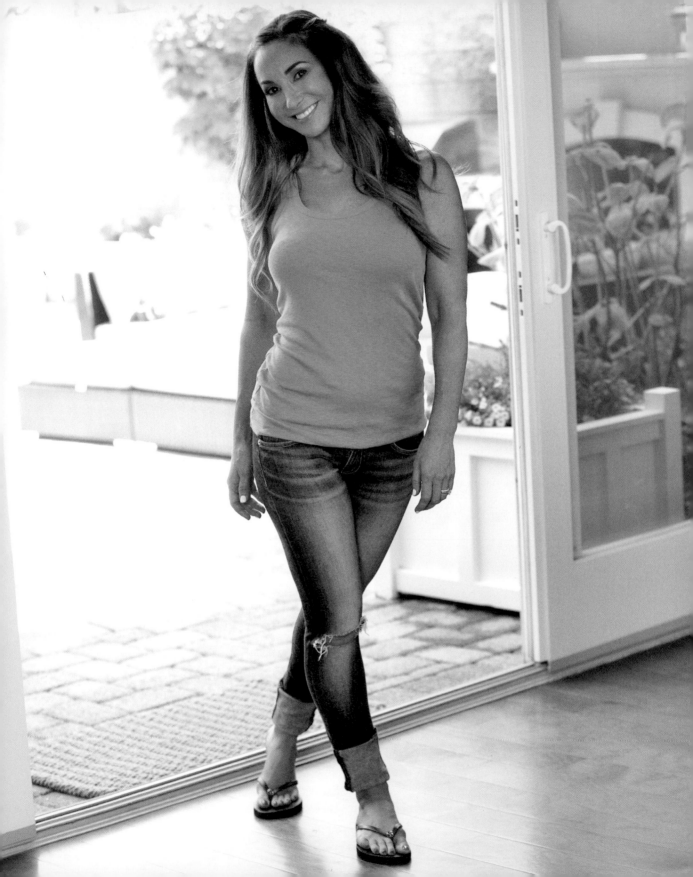

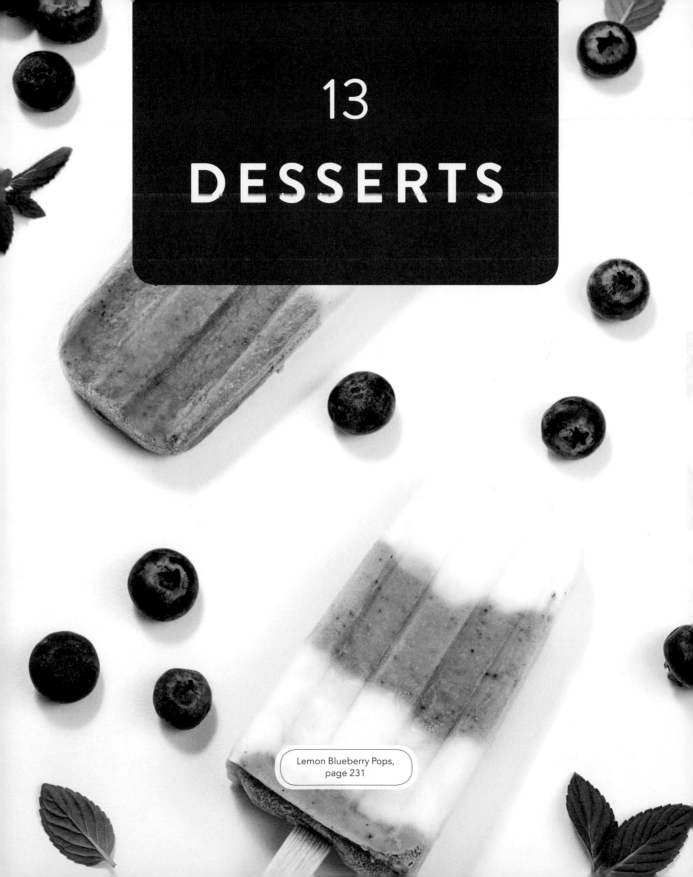

13
DESSERTS

Lemon Blueberry Pops,
page 231

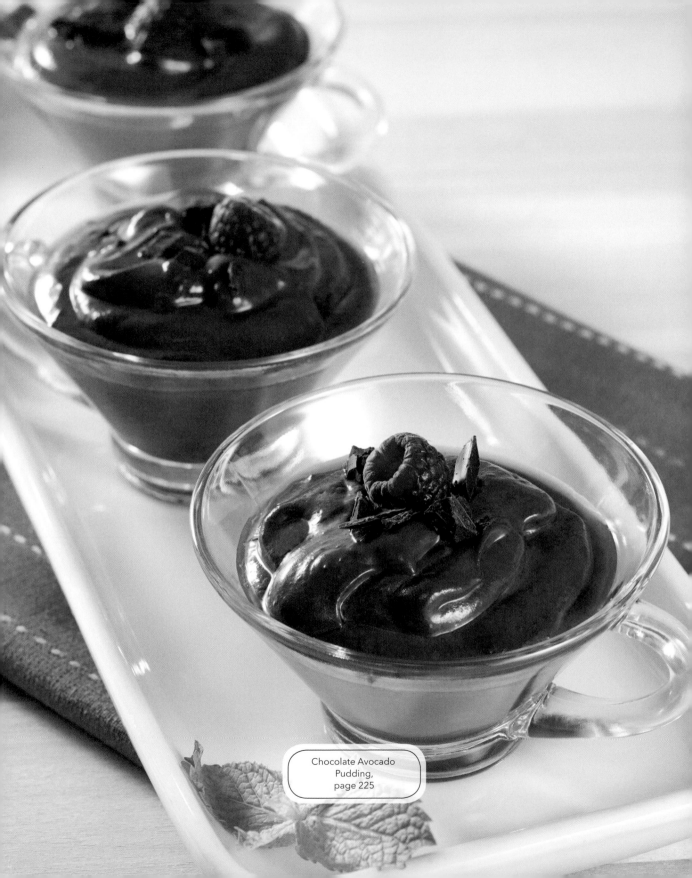

Chocolate Avocado
Pudding,
page 225

CHOCOLATE AVOCADO PUDDING

SERVES 4 (serving size: about ⅓ cup)

A chocolate lover's guiltless pleasure. Let your kids guess what the secret ingredient is—they'll never know there's nutritious avocado in it.

Ingredients:

1 ripe avocado
1 cup unsweetened almond milk
4 tablespoons natural
   non-alkalized cocoa powder
6 dates
½ teaspoon pure vanilla extract

Directions:

➤ Pureé all ingredients in a high-powered blender.
➤ You may add a little extra almond milk if needed to process. Pureé on high until smooth and creamy, scraping down the sides if necessary.
➤ Spoon into 4 bowls, or store in a covered container.

*You may add fruit or other topping of your choice.

Calories: 205/Calories from fat: 91
Fat: 10.1g, Protein 3.1g, Total carb: 30.7g, Fiber: 7.3g, Sugars: 21g, Sodium: 57mg, Vitamin A: 208mg, Vitamin C: 6mg, Calcium: 72mg, Iron: 1mg

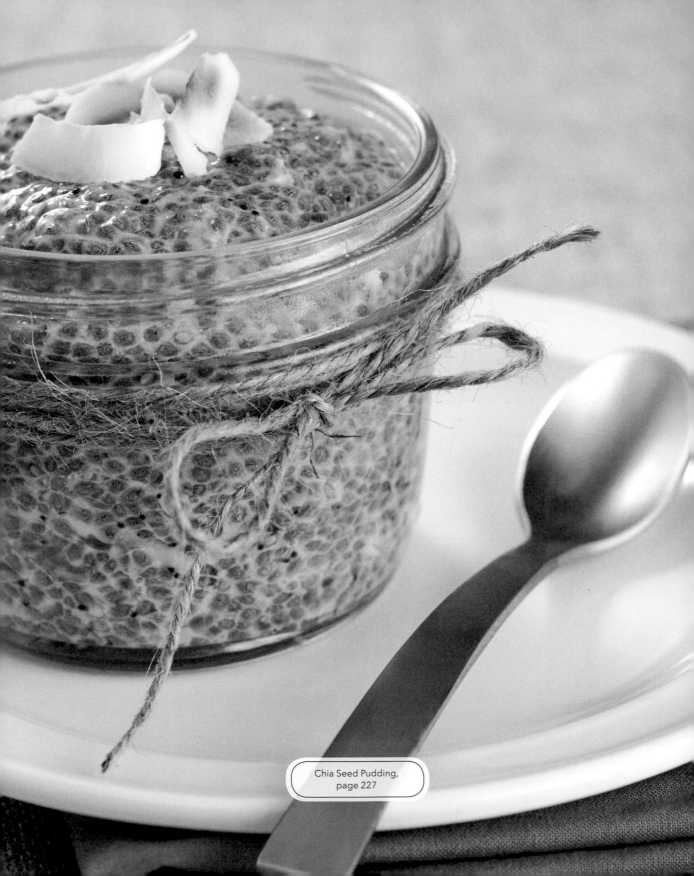

Chia Seed Pudding,
page 227

CHIA SEED PUDDING

SERVINGS: 6

Chia seeds are the Jump Start's answer to creamy, rich pudding: soak them and they'll magically transform any liquid into a pudding that's like tapioca but super healthy and filling. This protein-rich dessert is one that your friends will thank you for. (Add some fruit and nuts, and this makes a great breakfast, too!)

Ingredients:

- ¼ cup shredded, unsweetened coconut
- ⅓ cup chia seeds
- 1½ cup unsweetened coconut milk
- 2 tablespoons grade B maple syrup
- ½ teaspoon pure vanilla extract

Directions:

➤ Place all ingredients in a mason jar or any ½ pint-size jar with lid.

➤ Shake jar well and put into refrigerator. After 1 hour, take jar out and shake it again. Refrigerate at least four hours before eating.

Calories: 170/Calories from fat: 122
Fat: 13.5g, Protein: 2.7g, Total carb: 10g, Fiber: 3.5g, Sugars: 5g, Sodium: 18mg, Vitamin A: 5mg, Vitamin C: 0mg, Calcium: 62mg, Iron: 0.7mg

GRAIN-FREE COCO-NUTTY PORRIDGE

SERVES 2

Coconut and spice, warming to the soul and a great alternative for those who are cutting down on their processed carbs (that's you!). You could even eat this for breakfast or a half portion as a snack. Feel free to swap in another nut butter, such as cashew butter or sunflower butter and experiment with other spices such as cardamom, cloves, and ginger.

Ingredients:

- 2 tablespoons unsalted almond butter
- ¼ cup shredded unsweetened coconut
- 6 tablespoons unsweetened coconut milk
- ¼ teaspoon pure vanilla extract
- ½ teaspoon ground cinnamon
- Pinch of salt
- 1 teaspoon grade B maple syrup (optional)

Directions:

- ➤ Combine all ingredients in a bowl.
- ➤ Transfer to a saucepan and heat over low heat, stirring constantly until warmed through, about 3 minutes.

Calories: 310/Calories from fat: 235
Fat: 26.1, Protein: 5.2g, Total carb: 15.4g, Fiber: 4.7g, Sugars: 10g, Sodium: 84mg, Vitamin A: 2mg, Vitamin C: 1mg, Calcium: 49mg, Iron: 1.6mg

READY-TO-EAT CHOCOLATE CHIP COOKIE DOUGH

SERVES 8

You don't have to wait for these to bake! The best part of chocolate chip cookies is eating the dough—just spoon it right out of the bowl.

Ingredients:

- ½ cup packed almond flour
- ¼ cup tapioca flour
- 5 tablespoons cold, unsalted grass-fed butter
- 1 tablespoon agave nectar
- ¾ teaspoon pure vanilla extract
- 1 ounce chopped dark 85% chocolate
- Generous pinch of pink Himalayan salt

Directions:

➤ Combine all the ingredients except chocolate in a blender and blend until smooth. Stir in the chocolate and enjoy!

Calories: 149/Calories from fat: 109
Fat: 12.1g, Protein: 2g, Total carb: 8.6g, Fiber: 1.1g, Sugars: 3g, Sodium: 17mg, Vitamin A: 189mg, Vitamin C: 0mg, Calcium: 23mg, Iron: 0.7mg

BLUEBERRY YOGURT BITES

SERVING SIZE: 2 BITES (Makes 16 bites; serves 8)

Instead of relying on supermarket ice pops filled with sugar and colors not found anywhere in nature, make your own! It's easy, with no special equipment required, and you can swap in any type of berry you like. The yogurt and almonds add a protein boost, too!

Ingredients:

  1 cup plain Greek yogurt
  1 tablespoon coconut nectar
  1 cup fresh blueberries
  ½ cup chopped raw almonds
  16 popsicle sticks

Directions:

➤ Mix coconut nectar and yogurt together, stir in blueberries and chopped nuts.

➤ Place in a tray with molds in it such as a mini muffin tray or ice cube tray. After an hour, insert popsicle sticks.

➤ Freeze until firm, about 3 hours or overnight.

 TIP: Add a squeeze of lemon to any bowl of berries for a little zing.

Calories: 94/Calories from fat: 61
Fat: 6.7g, Protein: 3.8g, Total carb: 5g, Fiber: 1.5g, Sugars: 3g, Sodium: 9mg, Vitamin A: 22mg, Vitamin C: 2mg, Calcium: 46mg, Iron: 0.3mg

LEMON BLUEBERRY POPS

MAKES 6 pops

Blueberries are among the most powerful antioxidant fruits, and one of the tastiest, too. Pop one of these out from the mold and you're in for a treat. Now that's easy medicine!

Ingredients:

- 1 pint-size container fresh blueberries
- 1½ teaspoons fresh lemon zest
- 1 tablespoon fresh lemon juice
- 1¼ cups plain, full fat Greek yogurt
- 3 teaspoons agave nectar
- ½ cup unsweetened almond milk

Directions:

- ➤ In a blender, pureé the berries and 1 table-spoon of lemon juice until just smooth.
- ➤ In a small bowl, whisk together the yogurt, agave, milk, and lemon zest.
- ➤ In pop molds or paper cups, alternately layer 2 rounded tablespoons of the yogurt mixture and 1 tablespoon of the blueberry mixture. Swirl with a knife.
- ➤ Cover and freeze until firm, 4 hours or overnight.

Calories: 105/Calories from fat: 47
Fat: 5.2g, Protein: 3.6g, Total carb: 11.7g, Fiber: 1.3g, Sugars: 9g, Sodium: 29mg, Vitamin A: 90mg, Vitamin C: 6mg, Calcium: 0.1mg, Iron: 0.2mg

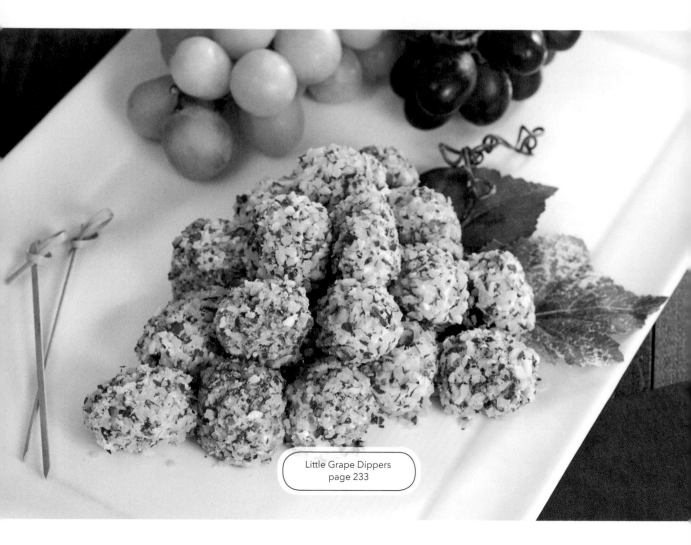

Little Grape Dippers
page 233

LITTLE GRAPE DIPPERS

SERVES 8

This cooling summer sweet looks adorable on the plate and is a great alternative to processed frozen desserts. Keep some handy in the freezer and reach for a few when you get the urge for ice cream.

Ingredients:

24 seedless grapes
1 8-ounce container Greek yogurt
2 teaspoons fresh lemon juice
1 teaspoon agave nectar
½ teaspoon pure vanilla extract
½ cup chopped almonds

Directions:

➤ Put each grape on a toothpick.
➤ Combine yogurt, lemon juice, agave nectar and vanilla in a small mixing bowl. Stir until well-blended.
➤ Crush the almonds until they are small enough to coat the grapes. Place the crushed almonds on flat surface on top of parchment paper.
➤ Dip the grapes in the yogurt dipping sauce, then roll them in the almonds and freeze.

Calories: 97/Calories from fat: 60
Fat: 6.6g, Protein: 3.7g, Total carb: 5.6g, Fiber: 1.1g, Sugars: 4g, Sodium: 9mg, Vitamin A: 22mg, Vitamin C: 1mg, Calcium: 47mg, Iron: 0.3mg

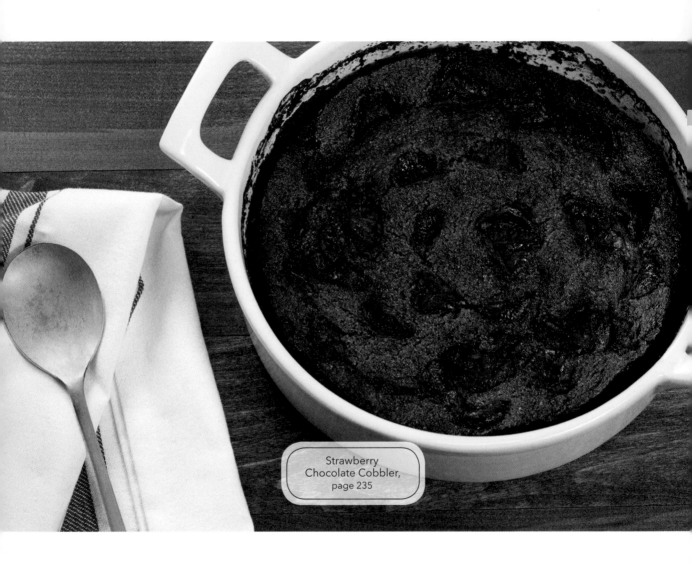

Strawberry
Chocolate Cobbler,
page 235

STRAWBERRY CHOCOLATE COBBLER

SERVES 8

Who doesn't love strawberries and chocolate? This cobbler tastes like an indulgence, but the ingredients' list proves that it's not. It can be served either warm or cold, and you can swap in any seasonal berry you like.

Ingredients:

- 6 tablespoons unsalted grass-fed butter
- ½ cup cocoa powder
- 1 cup coconut sugar
- 2 cups almond flour
- 2 teaspoons baking powder
- 1 teaspoon ground cinnamon
- 1 cup unsweetened almond milk
- 1 pint fresh strawberries, hulled and sliced

Directions:

- ➤ Preheat oven to 350 degrees.
- ➤ Combine the butter, cocoa powder, and ¼ cup of the coconut sugar in a 9x13-inch glass baking dish. Place in the oven for 3–5 minutes to melt the butter. Remove from the oven and stir until well-blended. Spread mixture out over the bottom of the baking dish.
- ➤ In a medium bowl, combine the flour, baking powder, cinnamon, and the remaining ¾ cup coconut sugar. Add the almond milk and stir until the mixture is smooth. Spoon over the melted butter mixture but do not stir. Scatter the strawberries on top.
- ➤ Bake for 45 to 55 minutes. Let stand for 15 minutes before serving.

Calories: 177/Calories from fat: 110
Fat: 12.3g, Protein: 4.2g, Total carb: 14.3g, Fiber: 2.4g, Sugars: 10g, Sodium: 80mg, Vitamin A: 144mg, Vitamin C: 10mg, Calcium: 69mg, Iron: 0.8mg

PART 3
FIT, HEALTHY, AND HAPPY FOR LIFE!

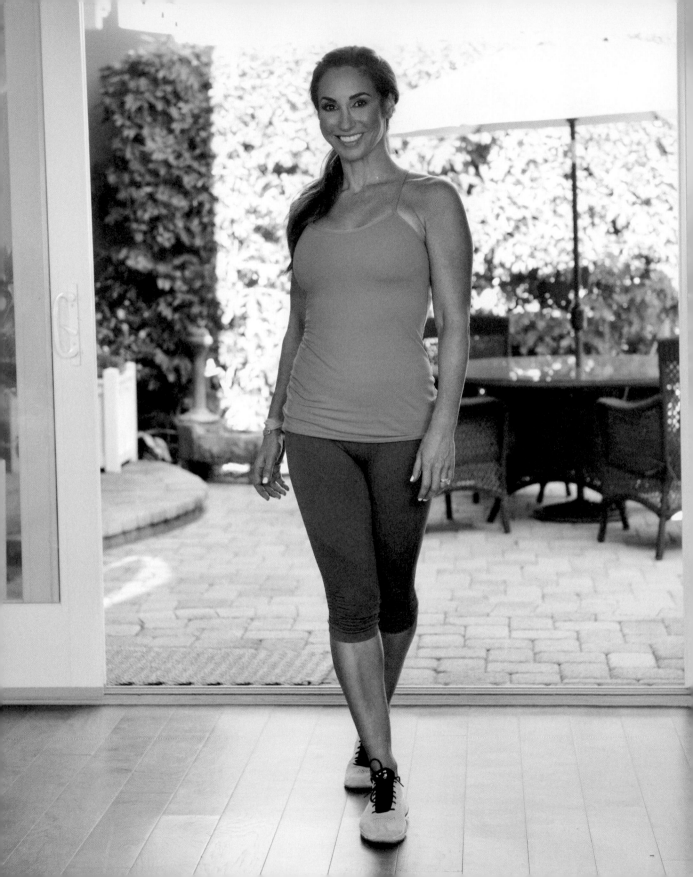

14

WORKING TOWARD STRONGER

"Working toward 'skinny' is discouraging, but working toward STRONGER is empowering—you will see!

NOW'S the time when we get to break a sweat, get those endorphins going, and have some fun! The single most important fitness habit you can learn is to walk and move your body daily. Keep in mind that it takes seventeen to thirty days to change an old habit and create a new one, so as you commit to my nutrition plan, it's equally important to commit to moving every single day until it becomes natural and part of your lifestyle. If you're not used to moving a lot, it may seem like a lot of change. But trust me—once you incorporate more movement into your daily life, your days won't be complete without it. A beginner might walk a mile, while someone in top shape may sprint for a minute; both require intensity, and both will give results. Just by doing what you're able to do now, know that you are progressing.

Now, when I talk about moving your body, it's not just about following an exercise plan. It's also about getting up and moving throughout the day. It's not just about looking lean and fit. You may be surprised to learn that sitting at a desk job can sabotage your health, posture, and fat-loss efforts.

SITTING IS THE NEW SMOKING

As human beings, we were not designed to sit in a car, behind a desk, or on the couch for so many hours a day.

In fact, the amount of time you spend sitting and not moving your body is a more important factor in fat- loss than exercise. Consider that for a moment. You know how so many people out there are constantly fixated on their workout routine? Yet so many of these people fail to realize that there is actually an even more important factor than their workout routine that they've given almost zero thought to—the amount of movement they're doing throughout the day.

It turns out that prolonged sitting can erase many of the benefits of exercise. New research shows that every hour that you sit erases between 8 and 16 percent of the metabolic benefits of your workouts! Do the math here! That means that even if you do an hour-long workout seven days a week, if you sit for ten hours a day, then you've just erased at least 80 percent of the metabolic benefits of that workout, and maybe well over 100 percent. One step forward, one step back. This is a recipe for working out hard and still spinning your wheels getting nowhere.

Prolonged sitting can even shorten your lifespan. One study, published in the *British Journal of Sports Medicine*, which included nearly 12,000 Australian adults, concluded that each hour spent watching television after the age of 25 reduces your life expectancy by nearly 22 minutes. By way of comparison with something you know is really bad for you, when the authors compared that reduction to smoking, they found that each cigarette reduces your life expectancy only by about 11 minutes. That's how sitting became the new smoking.

But there is good news—and it's called NEAT.

NEAT (NON-EXERCISE ACTIVITY THERMOGENESIS): IT'S NOT WHAT YOU DO AT THE GYM, BUT EVERYWHERE ELSE

In order to meet your fitness goals, you need to get off your butt, stand up, and move! I'm not talking about three or four times a week at the gym. Not twenty minutes or even an hour a day. If you want optimal health, amazing energy levels, a fast metabolism, and a lean body, you need to move throughout the day, every day. NEAT is basically all that movement that you do throughout the day just living your life—washing the car, running errands, climbing the stairs, walking down the street to the store, and even things like chewing gum, fidgeting, and tapping your feet. It is not what you do when you go to the gym like aerobics classes, riding the spin bike, or lifting weights. It's non-exercise activity.

NEAT is actually significantly more important than our exercise habits when it comes not only to fat-loss, but also for health, vitality, avoiding diabetes and many other chronic diseases, enhancing energy levels, speeding up our metabolism, and even prolonging our lives.

If you typically sit most of the day and are chronically low in energy and struggling to lose fat despite eating well and working out hard, NEAT is your answer. So get up and move again and again throughout the day, every day! The exercises offered in this chapter take 7 minutes—7 minutes!—and you can do them anywhere, since the only equipment you need is your own body. They'll get you to take a break from sitting, get the blood moving and the muscles working. Do that a few times a day and it will make a difference in the long run. You can think of it this way: 10 minutes per day of body weight exercises adds up to about 60 hours of working out over the course of a year. Sixty hours of working out definitely burns some calories, tones some muscle, and helps prevent that slow creeping weight gain over the course of the year!

PROGRESSION AND INTENSITY FOR REAL RESULTS

Intensity and pushing yourself with your fitness program is what will ultimately change your body. It doesn't take long hours in the gym to be healthy and have the body you desire. When I say the word intensity people often quickly jump to "that sounds too hard" or "I can't do that." But you can, because intensity is based on how it feels to you; it's different for each and every one of us. For example, walking up a flight of stairs could be very intense for somebody who weighs over 350 pounds and easy for someone at their goal weight. The key is just to push yourself. If walking up a flight of stairs is intense—good, then aim to do two flights the next time. Whether it's stairs, going for longer walks, or working on doing 25 pull-ups in a row, you just have to keep pushing yourself! Consider starting a fitness journal or using a fitness app and regularly noting how you are progressing.

Along those same lines, if you are doing something comfortable week after week, you aren't going to challenge your body or make any changes. For example, lifting the same light weights over and over again will not change your body after a certain point. Doing long cardio on stationary machines while talking on your cell phone or looking at a magazine will not change your body either. Yes, you may be watching the digital calorie counter slowly increase, but you are burning fewer overall calories than when you do strength training and HIIT (high intensity interval training) cardio. If you really enjoy working the machines, I'm not telling you to stop, but there are better uses for your time that will actually get you more measurable results, and isn't that what we all want—better results in less time?

Likewise, lots of reps with light weights will never get you to the next level. They are great for beginners getting started, but if you don't start progressing pretty soon, your body won't change. It's a great introduction to working out, and it gets the body burning calories and priming the muscles for more intense exercise down the road, but it will not drastically change your body, as the body will quickly adapt.

What you need to do is focus on pushing yourself, respecting where you are right now. Sweat more, get your heart rate up, and keep progressing every week. Sure, you can't do everything all at once, and your weights can't go up every week forever, but you get the point. You have to keep pushing for that extra rep, extra set, or more weight. If you are doing cardio, a good guide for working out with intensity is getting out of breath and getting your sweat on. Your workout should not be social hour, and you should not look cute at the end of your workout. Get in there, get to work, and give everything you have to your workout and watch your body change! Make yourself accountable with a friend, or record your progress in that fitness journal or an app like Toned by Natalie Jill. Go back to your vision board and remind yourself why you're doing this. Set daily goals. Pick new challenges to add to your day every day. Know that every step forward is a step in the right direction.

REACHING YOUR FITNESS GOALS WITHOUT WEIGHTS OR EXERCISE EQUIPMENT

Want to know the best kept secret to changing your body? Use your body! You can use your own body weight to change how your body functions, looks, and feels. All of my workouts—from beginning to advanced—require nothing more than your own body

weight. No weights, no equipment, no gym membership, and no commute. You can do everything in the comfort of your own home.

As a busy single mom, I didn't have a lot of extra time. So the time I did have, I wanted to make sure was spent wisely. So I tested all the exercise methods around, from the classic programs to the latest and greatest science-based fitness programs. I researched every study on training, weight loss, and personal fitness and found out exactly what the body does and doesn't need to burn calories and lose weight. But the weight loss wasn't the big discovery. I discovered that in literally just 10 minutes a day with no equipment, using just your own body weight, you can turn your body into a fat-burning machine and truly become physically fit. The following are seven of my favorite workouts.

SEVEN 7-MINUTE ANYWHERE WORKOUTS

What I really love about these workouts is that they can be done anywhere, anytime, without any specialized equipment. It's not even about counting reps or how many you do; it's more about pushing yourself, engaging the muscles you're targeting in each exercise, and progressing. If you're making these exercises more challenging as you go, you're good to go! Each of the exercises targets a specific area, while at the same time uses the body as a unit for a complete mini workout.

Remember, intensity and progression are what change our bodies. Do what is intense so you can progress! These workouts are designed to be very challenging, so don't be discouraged if you don't knock 'em out the first time through. The very act of working toward completing the exercises will help you change your body and get stronger. Do what you can, and push a little bit further every day. Work toward stronger! Use your fitness journal or app to record your progress and set goals.

Some basic tips:

- You don't need any equipment, though you'll be most comfortable in workout clothes and sneakers.
- Get in a quick warm-up—walking in place, swinging your arms—anything to get your body moving.
- These workouts are designed to be 7 minutes. Aim to work straight through the 7 minutes, but listen to your body and take breaks as needed. Each workout has stages for Beginner, Intermediate, and Advanced.
- Try to do one set a day. Feel free to mix up the exercises to create your own Jump Start fitness plan.
- For more inspiration, check out natalie jillfitness.com/dvds, nataliejillfitness .com/workout-calendar (a month of free workouts), and Youtube.com/natalie jillfitness.

1. GLUTE DEFINER

For each exercise:

BEGINNER: Start with 15 seconds of each with a 45-second rest.

INTERMEDIATE: Work up to 25 seconds of each with a 35-second rest.

ADVANCED: Work up to 45 seconds of each with a 15-second break.

GLUTE BRIDGE

Go into bridge position, lying on your back with your knees bent, arms at your sides, and hands and feet facing forward. Lift your hips up and hold, engaging your glutes. For this and all of the exercises in this sequence, press your lower back into the floor, keeping your abs and core tight and driving through your heels to really feel it in the targeted areas—your glutes, hamstrings, and thighs. You shouldn't feel this in your lower back.

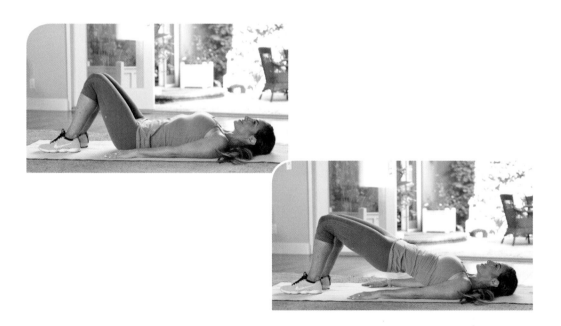

GLUTE BRIDGE UP AND DOWN

Lift your hips into bridge position and lower them back down. Repeat the up and down motion for counts of 2 (2 counts up, 2 counts down). Keep your abs and core stable.

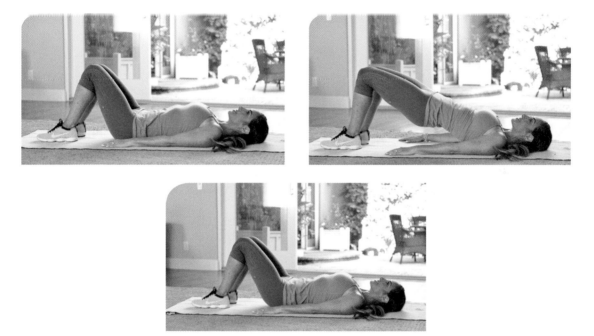

GLUTE BRIDGE OPEN AND CLOSE FROM UP POSITION

In bridge position with your hips up and abs and core tight, open and close your knees, engaging your inner thighs and core, and squeezing your glutes to create resistance (2 counts up, 2 counts down). Try to keep your core stable and avoid sinking into your lower back.

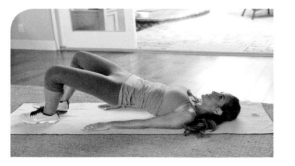
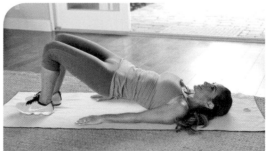

GLUTE BRIDGE UP AND DOWN WITH A SINGLE LEG

Lying on your back with your knees bent, lift your right leg up, keeping the knee slightly bent, then lift your hips up into bridge position and pulse it for 1 minute. Note that the movement is in the hamstrings and glutes, not the leg. Push through your heels and tuck your pelvis under so you don't feel it in your lower back (your back should not have a C curve in it), and keep your core super-tight.

Repeat with the left leg.

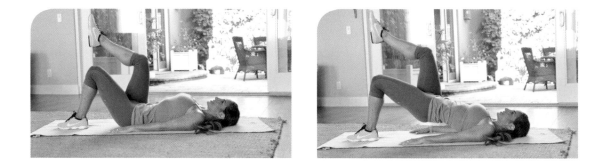

GLUTE BRIDGE SINGLE-LEG HOLDS

Lying on your back with your knees bent, lift your right leg, keeping the knee slightly bent. Lift your bottom, squeeze, and hold, engaging your glutes. Move to little pulses if this is too challenging. Repeat with the left leg. Remember to tuck in your pelvis and keep your core tight!

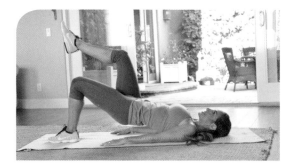

2. ARM TONER

TRICEP DIPS FROM SEATED POSITION

Start with your hands on the floor with your fingers facing forward. Walk your feet out so that your knees are at a 90-degree angle. Keep your abs and core tight. Dip your body down using your triceps and push back up. Every so often, do an alignment check and make sure those elbows are close to your body and not pointed outward.

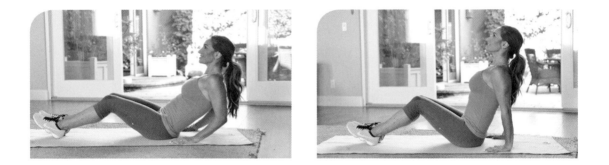

BEGINNERS: Start with 10 to 20 seconds of each with a 40-second rest.

INTERMEDIATE: Work up to 20 to 30 seconds of each with a 30-second rest.

ADVANCED: Work up to 30 to 45 seconds of each with a 15-second rest (it may feel relatively simple until the last 10 seconds or so).

TRICEP DIPS WITH GLUTES OFF THE GROUND

Start out in bridge position with your fingers pointed forward and feet flat on the floor. With your hips lifted and core tight, drop your elbows down and push back up. Rather than dropping your booty, think of this as slow and controlled from your arms. You don't need to speed through these. As with the previous exercise, every so often, do an alignment check and make sure those elbows are close to your body and not pointed outward.

BEGINNERS: Start with 10 seconds of each with a 50-second rest.

INTERMEDIATE: Work up to 30 seconds of each with a 30-second rest.

ADVANCED: Work up to 45 seconds of each with a 15-second rest.

Shake it out and take a quick break before the next exercise.

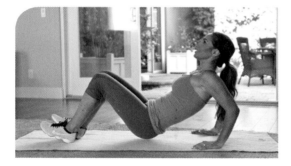 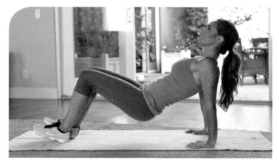

TRICEP SIT-THROUGHS

Start in bridge position with your hips lifted, palms and feet flat on the floor. Keeping your feet together, using your core and engaging your triceps, sit backward propped up by your hands by transferring your weight underneath you, and hold. Your butt will be hovering above the floor. Return to full bridge position and repeat. If this is too advanced, repeat one of the first two exercises. To make it more advanced, hold longer or do more.

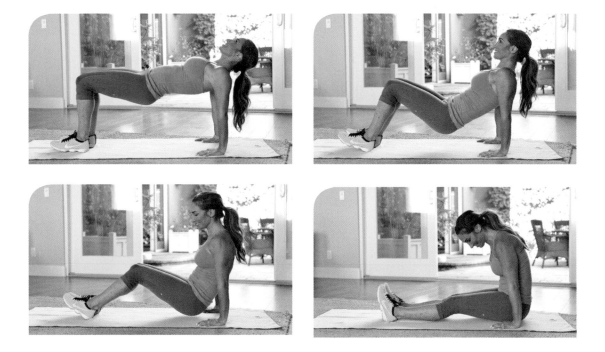

BEGINNERS: Work toward doing a single one. For this one, the act of working toward accomplishing 1 is progression!

INTERMEDIATE: Work up to doing 10 to 15 within 1 minute (to make it easier, touch your bottom down between each one).

ADVANCED: Work up to 45 seconds of these with a 15-second rest, keeping your bottom totally off the floor. You will feel this one in your core, triceps, and shoulders.

Rest for a full minute and shake out those arms.

TRICEP CRAB WALKS

Start in bridge position with your palms and feet flat on the floor. Suspend your weight on your hands and feet and "walk" forward and backward and side to side, focusing on your triceps muscles. Depending on available space, aim to walk forward and back and side to side 4 times. Remember to keep your hips lifted (they may tend to sink as you walk) and your core tight. Crab walk away!

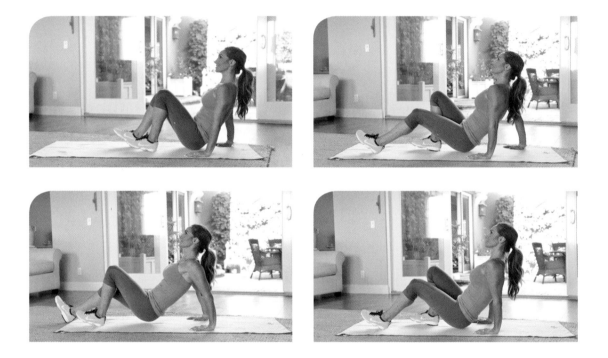

BEGINNERS: Start with 10 to 20 seconds with a 40- to 50-second rest.

INTERMEDIATE: Work up to 30 to 40 seconds with a 20- to 30-second rest.

ADVANCED: Work up to 1 minute, moving front, back, side to side. To advance even further, kick a leg up every 4 to 5 movements.

Rest and repeat.

TRICEP PUSH-UPS

From a push-up position, place your elbows close to your body, fingertips pointed forward. Lower yourself down to the push-up position and then back up. Keep those abs and core tight! Every so often, do an alignment check and make sure those elbows are close to your body and not pointed outward.

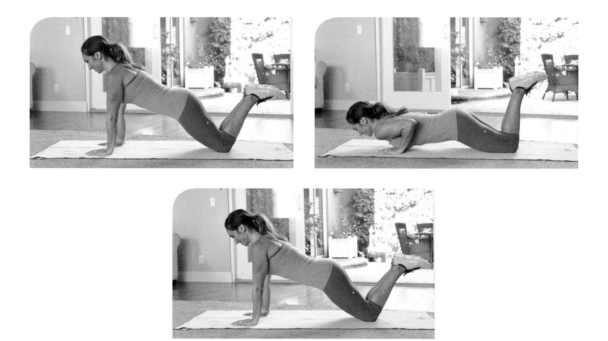

BEGINNER: Do these from your knees or standing with your hands on a sturdy chair. Work toward doing 5. Gradually increase each time you do this workout until you can do 15 from this position. You can go as slow as you need to!

INTERMEDIATE: Work up to push-ups from your feet with your elbows close in. Work toward 30 seconds with a 30-second break.

ADVANCED: Work up to a full minute of these. To add an extra challenge, do it again with one leg up for 30 seconds and the other leg up for another 30!

3. INNER THIGH SQUASHERS

PLIÉ SQUATS

In a standing position with your knees and toes pointed out, squat down into a plié squat, squeezing your inner thigh muscles. Hold for 2 counts, then come back up to full standing and hold for 2 counts and repeat. For an extra challenge (any level), hold your arms out in front of you while you do the exercise.

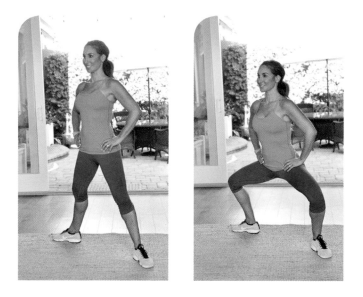

BEGINNERS: Start with 15 seconds with a 45-second rest.

INTERMEDIATE: Work up to 30 seconds with a 30-second rest.

ADVANCED: Work up to 60 seconds with a rest or no rest before moving to the next exercise.

PLIÉ SQUAT HOLDS

Go into a low plié squat position with your knees and toes pointed out, and hold. Your core and abs should be tight, with a long back and neck. For an extra challenge (any level), do bicep curls with your arms (create the resistance in your mind to make them challenging) while you do the exercise.

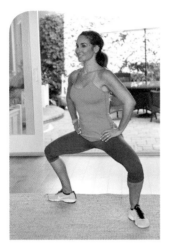

BEGINNERS: Start with 15 seconds with a 45-second rest.

INTERMEDIATE: Work up to 30 seconds with a 30-second rest.

ADVANCED: Work up to 60 seconds with a rest or no rest before moving to the next exercise.

PLIÉ SQUAT PULSE

In a low plié squat position with your knees and toes pointed out, add tiny pulses for 30 seconds. As with the previous exercise, keep your core and abs tight and your back and neck long. For an extra challenge (any level), hold your arms out to the sides or front while you do the exercise.

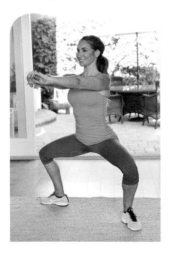

BEGINNERS: Start with 15 seconds with a 45-second rest.

INTERMEDIATE: Work up to 30 seconds with a 30-second rest.

ADVANCED: Work up to 60 seconds with a rest or no rest before moving to the next exercise.

TRAVELING PLIÉ SQUATS

Staying in a low plié squat position with your hands on your hips, walk yourself forward and back. Remind yourself to stay low! Keep your core and abs tight and your back and neck long. You'll really feel this in your glutes and thighs.

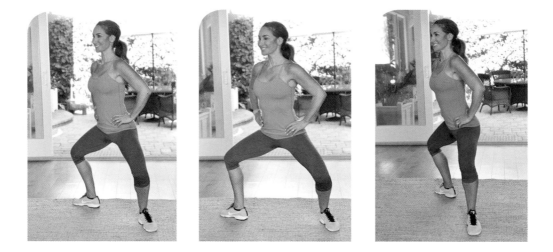

BEGINNERS: Start with 15 seconds with a 45-second rest.

INTERMEDIATE: Work up to 30 seconds with a 30-second rest.

ADVANCED: Work up to 60 seconds.

To challenge yourself further, take this sequence through 3 times.

4. LEG DEFINERS

HAMSTRING CURL, CROSS LEG OVER

Start lying face-down on the floor with your forehead resting on your mat or your hands and your arms bent at a 90-degree angle. Place your left foot on top of your right calf and lift your right leg, stopping at a 90-degree angle and lowering it back down. Use your left foot to create resistance on your right hamstring. Repeat and switch sides. All levels should work one side for 30 seconds, then switch sides and repeat for 30 seconds. Listen to your body. If 5 seconds is too challenging, stop there. You can also vary the resistance and pace.

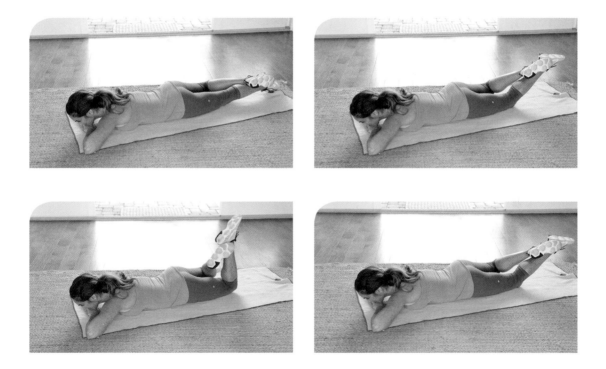

DONKEY SEQUENCE (5 MINUTES TOTAL)

Complete the entire sequence on one side, then repeat on the other side. To make it less challenging, do each exercise on both sides before moving on to the next.

DONKEY KICKS

Start with your forearms and knees on the floor and lift one leg behind you in a 90-degree angle. Make sure your foot is flat and flexed and push your foot toward the ceiling, squeezing your hamstrings and glutes. Keep your hips square and core tight. Try not to sink into your shoulders and keep your head and neck in line with your spine and looking straight down. Go slow on these—at least 2 counts up and 2 counts down.

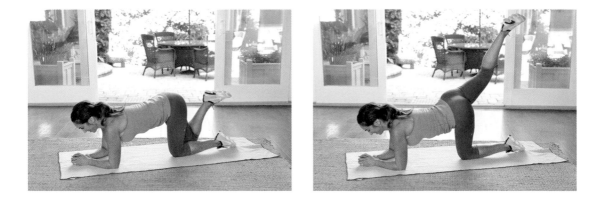

BEGINNER: Start with 10 seconds on each leg with a 35-second rest.

INTERMEDIATE: Work up to 30 seconds on each leg with a 30-second rest.

ADVANCED: Work up to 60 seconds on each leg with no rest.

STRAIGHT LEG KICKS

Start with your forearms and knees on the floor. Straighten out one leg and lift up and down, tapping your toe on the floor each time. Lift the leg all the way up in a slow and controlled manner using your glutes and hamstrings. Keep your head and neck in line with your spine and looking straight down.

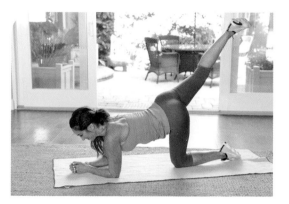

BEGINNER: Start with 15 seconds on each leg with a 30-second rest.

INTERMEDIATE: Work up to 30 seconds on each leg with a 30-second rest.

ADVANCED: Work up to 60 seconds on each leg with no rest.

DONKEY CURLS

Start with your forearms and knees on the floor. Straighten out one leg and bend your knee into a 90-degree angle, lifting your leg all the way in a slow and controlled manner using your glutes and hamstrings, then bring it back down to a straight leg and repeat. Make sure to keep your head and neck in line with your spine looking straight down.

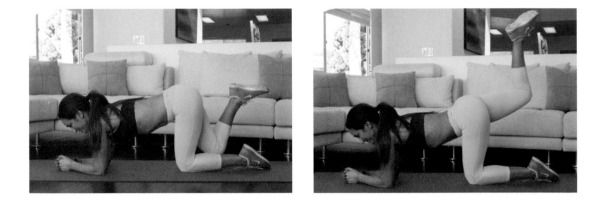

BEGINNER: Start with 15 seconds on each leg with a 30-second rest.

INTERMEDIATE: Work up to 30 seconds on each leg with a 30-second rest.

ADVANCED: Work up to 60 seconds on each leg with no rest.

Repeat the previous 3 exercises on the opposite side.

DONKEY LADDERS

Start with your forearms and knees on the floor. Lift your right leg behind you in a 90-degree angle with your foot flexed, and push your foot toward the ceiling, squeezing your hamstrings and glutes. Then get up onto your hands, and with that same leg, bring your knee in to meet your chest and push it straight back out. Go back on your forearms and continue to repeat the sequence. The transition between these movements is quick, so you'll be getting a little cardio in as you do it.

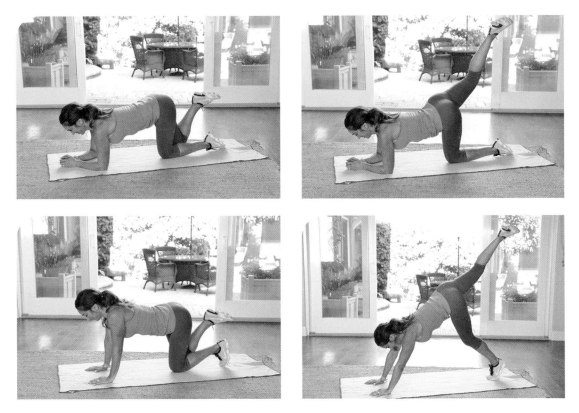

BEGINNER: Start with 5 reps with a 30-second rest.

INTERMEDIATE: Work up to 30 seconds with a 30-second rest.

ADVANCED: Do the Donkey Ladder Challenge.

Donkey Ladder Challenge: Alternate kicks up from the forearm-and-knee position and your hands and tippy toes. Start with 8 each, then 6, then 4, then 2, and finish with 10, up from your hands and tippy toes.

5. BACK AND GLUTE DEFINERS

WALL SITS

Start with your back pressed against a wall with your feet out in front of you, knees at a 90-degree angle, in a sitting position. Keep your core and abs tight, your back and neck long and straight. For balance, you have the option of reaching your arms out in front of you, resting on your hips or straight down by your side.

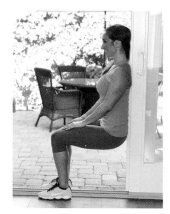

BEGINNER: Start with a 10-second hold. Walk it out for 30 seconds and repeat for another 10. Rest for 10 seconds before moving to the next exercise.

INTERMEDIATE: Work up to a 30-second hold.

ADVANCED: Work up to a 60-second hold.

SINGLE LEG UP WALL SITS

Start with your back pressed against a wall with your feet out in front of you, knees at a 90-degree angle, in a sitting position. Keep your core and abs tight, your back and neck long and straight. Lift your right leg out in front of you, keeping your arms out in front for balance, and hold for 30 seconds. Switch legs and hold for 30 seconds.

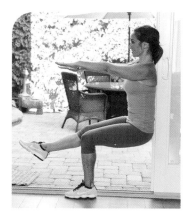

BEGINNER: Start with a 5-second hold for each leg. Walk it out for 30 seconds and repeat for another 5 seconds on each leg. Rest for 10 seconds before moving to the next exercise.

INTERMEDIATE: Work up to a 20-second hold for each leg with a 20-second shake-it-out and walk around.

ADVANCED: Work up to a 30-second hold for each leg.

LAT PULL-DOWNS AND RAISES AGAINST THE WALL

Start in a standing position with your back pressed against the wall, core engaged and your arms overhead. Using your own resistance, pull your arms down until your elbows are at your waist, squeezing your shoulder blades and using your back muscles to create resistance, and return to the starting position.

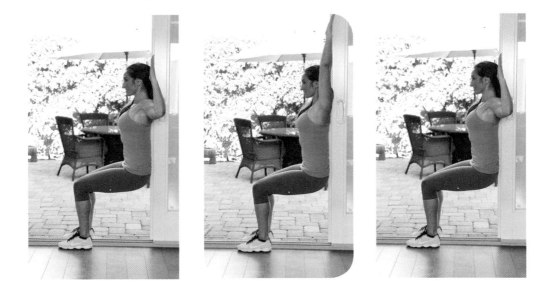

BEGINNER: Stand straight up against the wall (do not squat) and do the entire exercise from a standing position for 60 seconds.

INTERMEDIATE: Do 15 seconds from the standing position, then squat down to do 15 seconds from the squatting position.

ADVANCED: Work up to 60 seconds from the squatting position.

Walk around and shake it off for 1 minute, then repeat the entire sequence—wall squats, single leg wall squats, and lat pull-downs and raises against the wall.

6. FLAT BELLY DEFINER/CORE BUILDER

Note: This is a challenging workout for any level, and advanced is very challenging. The goal is to spend 7 minutes on it—even if you stay on the first exercise for the full 7 minutes. The suggested times are just suggestions. Go at your own pace.

It is critical that you do not arch your back while you do these exercises. Engage your core, suck your tummy in, bring your belly button into your spine, and create a flat back. If your form is not correct, you may feel pain in your lower back; when you are doing these correctly, they should feel good on your lower back. To make the plank exercises less challenging, tap your knee down to the ground and/or start from an aerobic step, chair, or bench, putting your hands on the platform and your toes on the ground.

FOREARMS PLANK HOLD

Start in standard plank position on your forearms and toes, and hold.

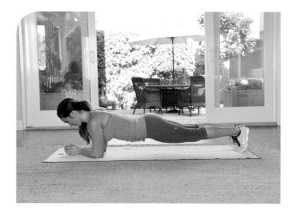

BEGINNER: Start with 5 seconds of each, 2 times within 1 minute.

INTERMEDIATE: Work up to 15 to 20 seconds of each with a 40-second rest.

ADVANCED: Work up to 30 to 45 seconds of each, with 15-second breaks and resting as needed.

PLANK TOE TAP SIDE TO SIDE

Start in regular plank position on your hands and toes. Tap your left toe to the side and return to starting position. Tap your right toe to the side and return to starting position. Continue, alternating sides, for 1 minute. Your core shouldn't really move; the movement is all in your legs.

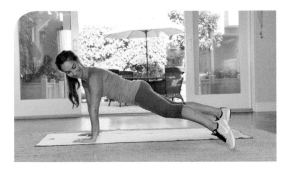

BEGINNER: Start with 5 seconds of each, 2 times within 1 minute.

INTERMEDIATE: Work up to 15 to 20 seconds of each with a 40-second rest.

ADVANCED: Work up to 30 to 45 seconds of each with 15-second breaks.

PLANK KNEE TO SAME-SIDE ELBOW

Start in regular plank position on your hands and toes. Bring your right knee in to meet your right elbow, then bring your left knee in to meet your left elbow. You really want to engage your obliques here.

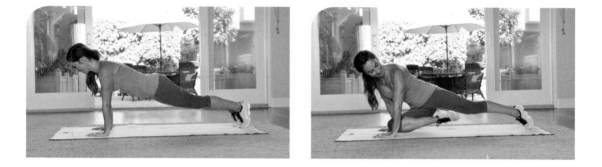

BEGINNER: Start with 5 seconds of each 2 times within 1 minute.

INTERMEDIATE: Work up to 15 to 20 seconds of each, with a 40-second rest.

ADVANCED: Work up to 30 to 45 seconds of each with 15-second breaks.

HAND PLANKS

Start in plank position on your palms and toes. Hold for 5 to 30 seconds depending on your level.

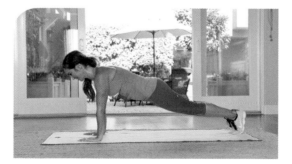

HAND PLANK KNEES TO OPPOSITE WRIST

Start in plank position on your palms and toes. Bring your right knee in to meet your left wrist and return to starting position. Bring your left knee in to meet your right wrist and return to starting position. Guide your hips as your knee meets your wrist. Continue for up to 30 seconds depending on your level, alternating sides. Always engage your core and don't let your hips drop down. This is a great exercise for your entire body, but you will feel it mainly in your abs, obliques, and shoulders.

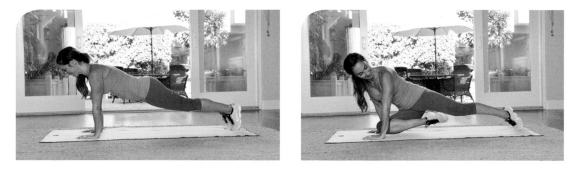

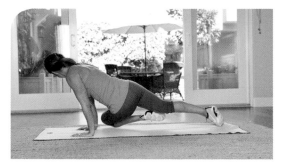

SIDE PLANK SEQUENCE

Go through the final three exercises below on one side, then repeat the entire sequence on the other side.

SIDE PLANK

Start in side plank position on your forearm and lift your hips. Hold.

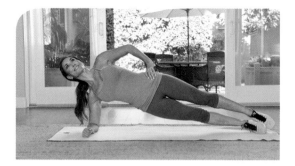

BEGINNER: Start with 5 seconds with a 25-second rest on each side. Keep your lower knee down.

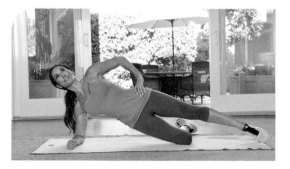

INTERMEDIATE: Work up to 15 seconds on each side with a 30-second rest.

ADVANCED: Work up to 30 seconds on each side working straight through.

SIDE PLANK LIFT, FOOT AND HAND UP

Start by lying on one side on the floor in plank position. Resting on your forearm, lift your outer leg and arm up and hold. Your arms will be shaped like the letter L.

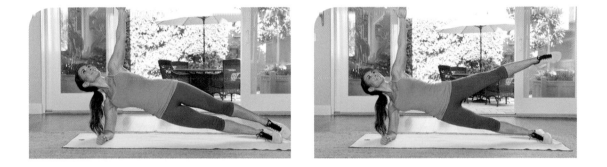

BEGINNER: Start with 5 seconds with a 25-second rest on each side. Keep your lower knee down.

INTERMEDIATE: Work up to 15 seconds on each side with a 30-second rest.

ADVANCED: Work up to 25 seconds on each side with a 5-second rest.

SIDE PLANK TUCK UNDER

Start in side plank position with one arm straight out. While twisting at the waist, take that arm and curl it under your body.

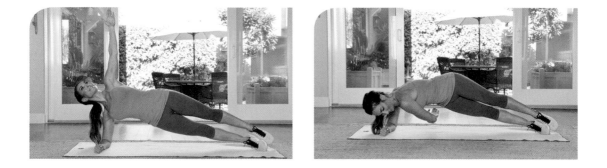

BEGINNER: Start with 5 seconds with a 25-second rest on each side. Keep your lower knee down.

INTERMEDIATE: Work up to 15 seconds on each side with a 30-second rest.

ADVANCED: Work up to 25 seconds on each side with a 5-second rest.

7. FULL BODY COMBO

Beginner and Intermediate: Pick 7 of your favorite exercises from the earlier workouts for a custom complete body workout.

Advanced:

HAND PLANK WITH CRISSCROSSED LEGS

Get into a hand plank position with your core tight and legs wide. Open up your left arm while, simultaneously, kicking your right leg through so your legs are crisscrossed. Aim for a 15-to-30 second hold and switch sides.

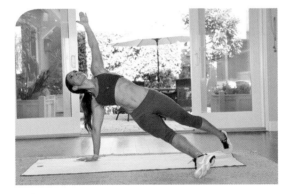

KNEE-TO-ELBOW HOLDS

Starting out on your right forearm plank position, bring your left knee to your left elbow, hold for 30 seconds, rest for 30 seconds, then switch sides.

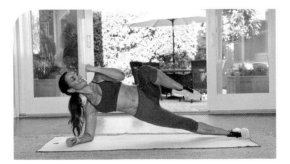

SINGLE LEG GLUTE BRIDGE

Lying on the ground with your arms alongside and your toes and fingers pointing forward, lift your butt off the ground, kick up one leg, and bring it back down. Use your triceps and stationary leg, driving through the heel, to get you there. Work up to 1 minute on each leg.

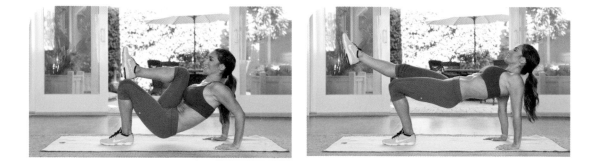

REVERSE BRIDGE HOLDS

From the previous position, with your butt off the ground, hold for 5 seconds, then take it back down and repeat. Do as many as you can in 1 minute.

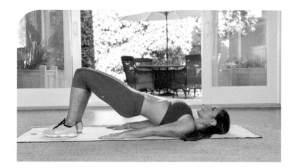

SIDE PLANK REACH AND TOUCH

From a side plank position, take it elbow to knee, working up to 30 seconds on each side with a 30-second rest between sides.

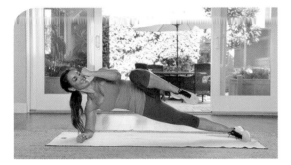 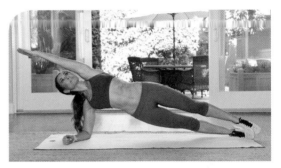

THE CORRECT WAY TO DO A PLANK

A plank is the #1 exercise to help develop your core! The core is the whole center of everything; it is the foundation of your body and what holds everything together. A strong core impacts everything you do! Here's how to do a perfect plank:

1. Start out on your forearms and toes.
2. Keep everything tight, hold that stomach in, and squeeze your glutes.
3. Move from your forearms to your hands and hold it there. Aim for 1 minute, then shoot to hold for longer. Next, try a variation move like a side plank if you like.

TIP: Many people have a natural C-curve in their back; if that's you, you're really going to want to make sure your pelvis is tucked in and your lower back is flat. Do not arch your back. It may look more flattering to arch your back, but don't give in to vanity!

THE POSTURE SQUEEZE

OUR sedentary lifestyle—sitting all the time and being on the computer or phone for hours on end with your head tipped forward—is not doing our posture any favors. For healthy posture, we need to get up and move often throughout the day! This is a great quick fix for posture that you can do anytime, anywhere. Here's what to do:

1. Stand with your knees and toes pointed outward, shoulder-width apart.
2. Clench your glutes (butt muscles).
3. Tighten your core.
4. Stand up tall, pull your shoulders back, and keep your chin high.
5. Keeping everything tight, take a few deep breaths, and enjoy how this feels.

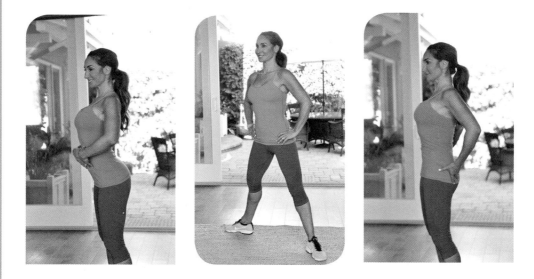

You should feel taller, with your lower back relaxed, and you should be able to breathe better. You can do this exercise anytime you are standing up, and nobody has to know you are doing it! Do it any time you are waiting in line or standing up, and see how much better you feel.

HOW I BEAT IRREVERSIBLE BACK PAIN

At forty, when the thought of a workout went from motivating and exciting to making me think of pain, I knew I had a problem. Everything hurt my back: sitting, standing, sleeping, and working out made the pain unbearable at times. As intense as the pain was, I was determined to "fix it"!

I sought out orthopedic surgeons and had an MRI, which confirmed that I had severe arthritis in my lower back and two bulging discs. I guess all those years of wearing high heels and skipping my workout warm-ups were starting to catch up.

I began a series of doctors' appointments and came out with prescriptions for arthritis meds, pain meds, cortisone shots, and so on. I saw four physical therapists, three orthopedic surgeons, and two chiropractors. All told me the same thing: the arthritis is permanent.

So my mission began to find a natural way to stop the pain, and here's what I learned: you can't "get rid of" arthritis, but you can stop what is causing the pain. It is not actually the arthritis or disc causing the pain; it's other imbalances around it causing you to feel pain where the issue is. You need to fix other areas of your body to get around those muscle imbalances.

I came to the conclusion that my workouts were no longer working for me. I had gotten into a comfort zone and was in denial that they were now wrong for me. I had to accept this fact and take on the challenge to re-learn the exercises and corrective circuits. I am diligent about doing these now, and there are some exercises that I can never do again or my back pain will instantly flare up.

Another thing I learned: I had abs, but my core was not functional. When I tried to do traditional exercises like crunches, my back would flare up because I had absolutely no core strength. It's amazing how quickly this can change with practice. This was my approach:

1. Body weight exercises: I moved primarily to exercises utilizing my own body weight and really worked to develop my core. No sit-ups (those only work the abdominal muscles), but true core strength, meaning your entire midsection (like a tree trunk). I'm not suggesting you start at that point, but it's something to work toward. It might seem like you are going backward at first, but if you stick with it, you will see amazing results!

2. Corrective circuits: I started doing corrective circuits, which help to activate muscles you haven't been using and help you calm down and release the muscles that are tight and overactive. As an example, my glutes were underactive, which is common in women. My quads and lower back were picking up the slack. Now I do a full corrective circuit to activate my glutes prior to my workouts so that my glutes pull their weight and take additional strain off my quads and lower back.

3. No more machines: My old workouts put too much stress on my lower back. I no longer do the weighted leg presses that used

to be a staple in my workout. Instead, I do exercises that keep my core engaged, using all of my muscle fibers. No more machines for me, as I find they are too isolating and can lead to the creation of muscle imbalances.

4. Anti-inflammatory diet: I also decided to take my diet up a notch and get diligent about adding key anti-inflammatory foods to my diet including the removal of grains and dairy. If you have an inflammatory disease, this is something you might want to look into.

Today my back is no longer in constant pain. It is not 100 percent fixed, but it is now limited to a few hours of pain a few days a month. My workouts are back to being intense, and I am once again changing and improving my body without the added fear and result of pain!

LISSA'S TRANSFORMATION:

From Creeping Weight Gain to Roller Derby Ready

Watching the weight creep up: I've always been active, but for some time I had been relying on my younger days when I could eat whatever I wanted without worrying about the consequences. Boy, the weight sure crept up on me. Too much eating on the go and mindless snacking were taking their toll. I work in law enforcement [dealing] with some pretty intense cases, so I need to be physically fit for my own safety, and I was starting to push those limits. I'm a pretty daring person, and I learned how to roller skate when I was forty-two just so I could play roller derby. Roller derby requires a lot of athleticism—just what I needed to get my body back on track.

Getting on board, but not 100 percent: Finding Natalie Jill's program online helped me get back on track. I immediately loved the message. I also loved that Natalie Jill was in her forties, had a child (I have three kids and two grandkids), and still looked amazing. Of all the fitness coaches out there, Natalie was the only one I felt a connection with. The twenty-year-old coaches are great, but who doesn't look great at twenty? When I was in my twenties, I was modeling and felt fantastic, but it was easy to maintain back then. I started my first Natalie Jill challenge in the beginning of the new year. I was onboard, but I still wasn't putting in 100 percent. I would cheat here and there, but still I was making some good progress. And then I had a big setback.

My pity party: I had been playing roller derby for two years, and I was doing great. I was trying hard to focus on eating clean, drinking water, and working out. Then one day in the spring I broke my leg during practice. I had a complete pity party and started to eat poorly again. I reverted back to all my

LISSA BEFORE

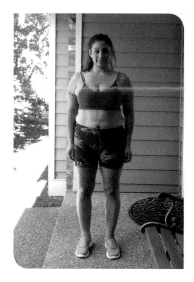
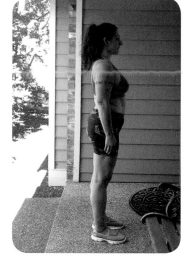
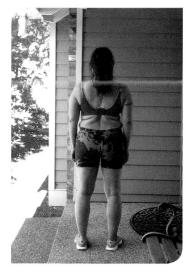

LISSA AFTER

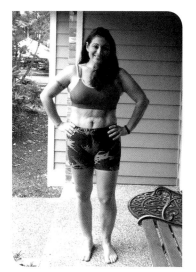
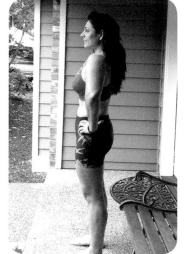
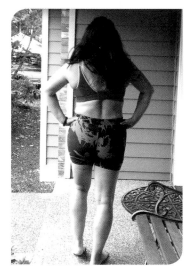

bad habits and gained pretty much all of the weight I'd lost. I felt horrible—I was fatigued and had headaches all the time. I knew I needed to get with the program, because my health was suffering.

Getting back on track: After I had had enough of feeling sorry for myself, that summer I told myself that this time I would really commit to a second challenge. I began eating well again, and for fitness I started with my upper body and core, then slowly brought back cardio and legs. Natalie Jill has so many workouts to choose from that I found there really was no excuse for not working out. I can't say that I've been perfect, but I feel wonderful—my energy level is back and I don't feel that constant fatigue that I was dealing with before.

A sign that I was doing things right: About five weeks into the challenge, I had guests staying with me, and I fell off a little.

I immediately got a headache, the first headache I had since starting the challenge. I used to get headaches every single day, but I hadn't had a single one during those five weeks. I wasn't drinking enough water, and I wasn't eating like I was supposed to, so this headache was telling me something. By following the program, not having a headache had become my new normal!

Getting back on my skates: For my second challenge, I really did my homework. I made a vision board. I did a lot of reading about health and nutrition. I didn't just follow the rules; I really educated myself so I would have an understanding of why I needed to stay away from processed foods. Doing that has made it easier to make better choices. I've lost about 10 pounds so far and I feel great. While I'm waiting for my doctor to clear me for full contact, I'm thrilled to be back on my skates and playing with my roller derby team again!

15

MAINTAINING YOUR RESULTS:
TO INFINITY AND BEYOND!

"Be happy . . . Be healthy . . . Be fit!"

MAINTENANCE. This seems like the hard part, right? You've "deprived" yourself of so much over the past seven days . . . or have you?

If you are like a lot of people I work with, at this point you love the way you feel, your clothes are starting to fit better, and you want to keep going! You feel lighter. You have accomplished something, and you are happy about it! You might not be at your goal in seven days, but you like the path you are on and the direction you are headed. You like this "new you" and don't see yourself going back. Some of you have made great strides toward achieving your end goal but have more to do.

This is decision time. Think about what your diet has looked like over the past week. Has it really been that grueling? It may have been hard at first, but it's likely you've started to develop patterns and habits that will allow you to continue on the same path and further your progress.

One important thing to remember is that something is always better than nothing. It doesn't matter how busy you are—anybody can do 7 or 10 minutes of body weight exercises every day. It takes no equipment, no travel, nothing but a small amount of floor space and a few minutes of your time. Just a few minutes over the course of a year can really add up.

As far as nutrition goes, it doesn't take any more time to make good choices than it takes to make poor choices. If all else fails or you're on the road and you have to eat "bad," just make the better choice, watch your portion sizes, and do the best you can. As you saw in Chapter 7, you can do this even at a fast-food restaurant.

Here's one of the keys to success: really understanding the benefits of continuing on and not slipping back into old habits. Yo-yo nutrition and fitness can actually be more detrimental to the body than not participating in a program at all, so please understand the importance of staying on a positive path toward long-term health and wellness. Here are some tips to make this happen:

Commit to Happy, Healthy, and Fit: An old saying goes: "Put the body in motion and the mind will follow." When you commit—really commit—to change, you can achieve anything.

Prepare Yourself: Keep your kitchen stocked with the basics so you don't find yourself scrambling with no good meal options. Take the time to plan your weekly grocery shopping and meals. Once you get into the habit of it, you'll find the process super-streamlined. To make maintenance easy away from home, keep your home, car, and office well-stocked with healthy options so you never have the excuse to binge on unhealthy snack foods. Going out to dinner? Check your options online before you get to the restaurant. Remember, there is nothing wrong with eating something before you get there. That way you aren't "starving" and ready to devour the breadbasket or other finger foods sitting there to tempt you. It is a lot easier to make the better decisions when you aren't that hungry.

Traveling? Check online or call your hotel ahead of time and find out what fitness options are available, whether it's a hotel gym or fitness center nearby. If you're going to be out in the country, research nature trails and bring your hiking boots. A little bit of effort and forethought go a long way in program maintenance. You can build your own program out of the 7-minute exercises in the previous chapter, or check out my DVDs (see page 287) or my YouTube channel, Youtube.com /nataliejillfitness.

Remind Yourself: Remember those goals you wrote out on pages 22 to 23? Revisit them. Then go to your vision board (pages 24 to 26) and remind yourself of the original reasons you decided to lose weight and get in shape. These mental weigh-ins are important, as they create accountability.

Remember the Majority Rules: What you do most of the time is what matters. Do you eat healthful, clean, and unprocessed foods at the majority of your meals? If you *do* eat properly most of the time, then the little bit that you choose not to won't be the end of the world for your health or physique. However, if you eat poorly more often than not, then you're fooling yourself. Majority rules, and your habits are clearly reflected in your body. That said, if you can't get rid of those last few pounds, then you *do* have to look at dialing things in and taking it up a notch for a bit so you can get there.

Work for It: When I *really* want a substantial treat, I work for it! Recently, I found myself craving pizza (the gluten-free kind). Instead of ordering it or driving to pick it up, I walked for it. Yup—five miles round trip—and by the time I got there and ordered the pizza, a small slice sufficed. And there was no guilt because I'd walked those five miles to get it.

Repeat Yourself: After you hit your weight-loss and fitness goals, you may start to get a little lazy, slip a little, and go back to older habits. If your waistline and weigh-ins tell you that is the case, just repeat the 7 Day Jump Start. There are plenty of recipes to keep you happy for another week or more. You'll get yourself right back on track in no time! I have lots of people who go back and do the seven days every couple of weeks just because it helps them stay on track.

Be Human: Being superhuman is for superheroes. Thinking you can use willpower through everything, like eliminating cravings and eating perfectly forever, is ridiculous. You have to live your life. This is the ebb and flow, yin and yang of life. If you live only on celery and fish, you will relapse eventually, and it will be ugly. Be human, enjoy your life—but keep the majority of your diet clean and healthy. Remember, it is about a lifestyle. By doing the right things right *most* of the time, it allows you to enjoy a treat every now and then.

Don't Beat Yourself Up: If you fell off track or are starting to go back to bad habits, don't beat yourself up; just move on and continue to work toward your goals.

Don't Compare Yourself to Others: Focus on competing with yourself to make progress. As soon as you start comparing yourself to others, you're more likely to get discouraged and fall off track. Focus on getting yourself healthier, better, and stronger and improving yourself daily. Working toward skinny can be discouraging. Working toward stronger is empowering.

Find Support to Get Past Your Hurdles: We all have potential challenges. Each of us, whatever we're striving toward, will face hurdles along the way. From the aroma of baked goods, to the group of friends getting together at a fast-food joint, to the temptations on the table at office meetings, it seems that potential hurdles are everywhere for those of us trying to make a lifestyle and way-of-eating change. But don't cave! Look for a support group in your community or on social media. Make sure the group has positive energy and makes you feel good about yourself.

Recruit Friends: Share with your friends what you've learned and get them onboard. Form a team with others to help keep you accountable.

Think Addition, Not Subtraction: This is a lifestyle, not a diet, so don't think about what you can't do. Instead, think about what you can *add* to your life every day—and I'm not just talking about veggies. Think positive reinforcement.

Change up Your Veggies: One of my followers committed to trying a new green every week. Why not try the Chopped Kale Salad (page 146) this week and next week the Asian Salad (page 141) featuring Napa cabbage?

Try a New Recipe: You've got 82 of them to choose from right here in this book!

Each of us has a different reason for wanting to reach our ideal weight: better health, self-esteem, or even winning a bikini contest! But each of us gets the same result: improved energy, vitality, health, and well-being. How will losing weight change *your* life? Allow yourself to imagine it. Get a clear picture of the future you. Now, go toward your goal. Do the work, follow my advice, and you'll get there. In addition, I've found that bringing the same goal of "unprocessing" to other areas of your life can have incredible benefits.

Think of it this way: I'm advising you to stick to what's real, not only with your food choices, but with every choice you make in your life. Now that's a game-changer! When I hit rock bottom, I realized that what I needed more than anything else was to get real with myself. And you know what? That turned out to be the best thing that could have happened to me. Why? Because in those raw, unprotected, authentic moments, my new career and my calling were found. Yours can, too!

KELLY'S TRANSFORMATION:

From Fast-Food Eating to "Feeling Good in My Skin"

Starting at my heaviest weight ever: When I found Natalie Jill's program, I was at my heaviest weight aside from my pregnancy weight. I wanted to feel as beautiful as my husband tells me I am, and I wanted to be comfortable in my own skin.

Looking for accountability: Discipline and accountability were what I needed to get myself on track. And I needed something that would work fpr a full-time working mother of two. I was drawn to Natalie Jill's Jump Start because it was put together so well, and I love that it is more than a diet but a lifestyle change. The program seemed like something I could stick with. I'm an extremely picky eater, and I have really struggled to get away from processed junk food.

Breakfast became important: I had never eaten real breakfasts; a granola bar at my desk was typical for me. Now I'm enjoying scrambled eggs, turkey sausage, cantaloupe, and other healthy real-food options. Eating a good breakfast gets me off to a good start and keeps me motivated to go the rest of the day unprocessed. No more hamburger and French fries for lunch. And no more drive-throughs

KELLY BEFORE

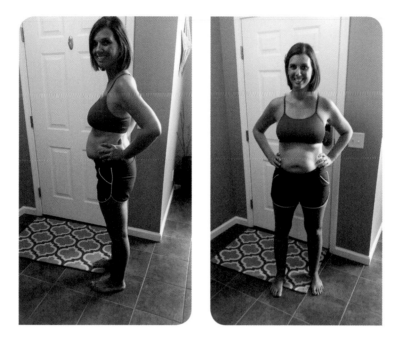

KELLY AFTER

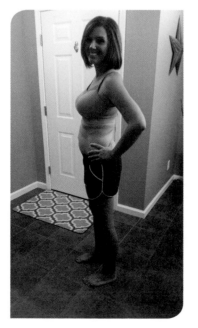
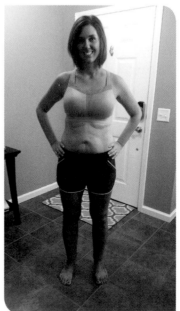

with the family for dinner. It was easier to swap in meal planning for fast-food eating than I thought. Plus, I've found a gluten-free bread that I like, so I can still make turkey sandwiches to bring to work. I add some fruit and cottage cheese, and that's all I'll need to make it through to dinner.

Becoming conscious of my food and my mission: I've become really good about looking at food labels and choosing all-natural food over food that's processed. And I know now that if I ever get off track, it's easy to get right back on. At first I thought I could skip the vision board, but when I finally did the work, it made all the difference in achieving my goals. In the past, I'd never really been good about exercise, but now I'm enjoying Natalie's workouts, and I really like her YouTube videos.

Visible changes: I have gotten rid of so much of the bloat, and my stomach has gone down quite a bit. I can fit more comfortably into my pants—without the muffin top. I've lost close to 10 pounds! My goal was to wear a bikini for my ten-year wedding anniversary trip. Life got in the way, and we were unable to take the trip, but it didn't really matter because that vision gave me great motivation for sticking with the program. I used to wear shorts and a T-shirt over my swimsuit, and I was always so self-conscious about that. But I've gotten to the point where I no longer need to cover myself up, and I am so pleased! I feel good in my skin.

Not a diet but a way of life: I've gone through lots of different diets, but I don't think of the Jump Start as a diet but a way of life—it's not something that I have to do but that I *want* to do. Natalie's program is so easy to follow, and I can tell that she truly cares about helping others. Knowing that has made all the difference.

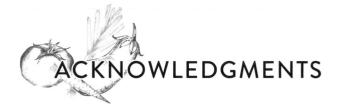ACKNOWLEDGMENTS

FIRST off, I want to thank Renee Sedliar and the team at Da Capo Press, including John Radziewicz, Kevin Hanover, and Kate Burke, for their support and contagious energy as we took this vision and made it a reality. Writing a book is an amazing experience and a very involved process. This book would not have been possible without the professional guidance from the following people (in no particular order): Celeste Fine, Natalie Minh, Mandy Schaffer, Ellen Scordato & her team, Leda Scheintaub, Julie Grimes, John Maas, and Justin White.

In addition to the professionals that made this book possible, there were the friends and family that supported and helped me along the way. Thank you to my "adopted mom," as I call her, Mindy Marinos, for your endless help through the entire process. Thank you to Liana Hunt, Lauren Reid, Wendy Chermak, and Nikki VanWinkle for keeping things on track and your attention to detail. Thank you Ari Whitten for always challenging me to learn more and to my mom who continues to believe in me and encourage me to achieve new goals, and thank you to Kim Bauman for encouraging me to always "slow down" and enjoy the process

To the best of friends, Michelle Conner, Jan Adams, and Shelli Pelly who have believed in me and encouraged me throughout this entire project. Thank you for always being there for me and for being the best of friends that I could ask for.

To David Josza, Chalene Johnson, and Tamilee Webb for being the most amazing mentors I could have ever known and learned from. You three have impacted my life more than you will ever know or understand. You believed in me at times when I doubted myself and empowered me to put my best self forward and go for my goals.

To Brett Hoebel, Lewis Howes, Casey Ho, and Keri Glassman who shared endless tips with me about publishing a book.

A SPECIAL thank you to my mom, Lorraine Levin, for always encouraging me to go for my dreams and to my husband, Brooks

Hollan, and my daughter, Penelope. You two are my world, what I live for. Your support and encouragement on this book and your belief in me is the greatest motivation I could ask for.

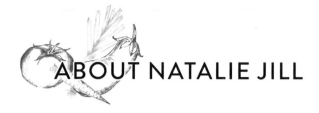

ABOUT NATALIE JILL

NATALIE left a very successful career in corporate America to follow her passion for health and fitness. She now helps people across the globe reach their health, fitness, and business goals. As a Licensed Master Sports Nutritionist and functional fitness trainer, Natalie leveraged the power of the Internet, and in a short amount of time has been able to help hundreds of thousands of people worldwide get in shape and be their best selves. In the process, she created a globally recognized brand with over two million social media followers worldwide. Although many see Natalie Jill as a fitness and nutrition expert, she is increasingly garnering attention for her ability to help others create and define their own brand in an online space. In health and fitness or in business, Natalie's mission is no less than to bring out the best in you!

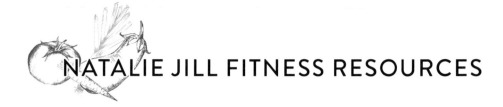

NATALIE JILL FITNESS RESOURCES

WWW.NATALIEJILLFITNESS.COM

NATALIE JILL FITNESS DVDS

www.nataliejillfitness.com/dvds
Natalie Jill 7 Day Jump Start™ Total
   Bodyweight Beginner
Natalie Jill 7 Day Jump Start™ Rev4
   Bodyweight Intermediate
Natalie Jill 7 Day Jump Start™ Building
   Abs Advanced
Natalie Jill 7 Day Jump Start™ Total
   Bodyweight Advanced

STRONGER TOTAL BODY ADVANCED WORKOUT PROGRAM

www.nataliejillfitness.com/stronger

MIND BODY ACADEMY

8-week module training on how to achieve
   real, lasting results not just in weight
   but in life

www.nataliejillfitness.com/programs/
   mind-body-academy/

FREE MONTHLY WORKOUT CALENDAR

www.nataliejillfitness.com/workout-calendar/

BUSINESS BUILDING AND BRANDING

www.nataliejillfitness.com/biz/

SOCIAL MEDIA

Twitter: @nataliejillfit
Youtube: Youtube.com/nataliejillfitness
Pinterest: Pinterest.com/nataliejillfitness
Instagram: @nataliejillfit
Facebook: www.facebook.com/nataliejillfit

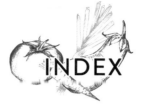

INDEX

METRIC CONVERSIONS

The recipes in this book have not been tested with metric measurements, so some variations might occur.

Remember that the weight of dry ingredients varies according to the volume or density factor: 1 cup of flour weighs far less than 1 cup of sugar, and 1 tablespoon doesn't necessarily hold 3 teaspoons.

General Formula for Metric Conversion

Ounces to grams	multiply ounces by 28.35
Grams to ounces	multiply ounces by 0.035
Pounds to grams	multiply pounds by 453.5
Pounds to kilograms	multiply pounds by 0.45
Cups to liters	multiply cups by 0.24
Fahrenheit to Celsius	subtract 32 from Fahrenheit temperature, multiply by 5, divide by 9
Celsius to Fahrenheit	multiply Celsius temperature by 9, divide by 5, add 32

Volume (Liquid) Measurements

1 teaspoon = ⅙ fluid ounce = 5 milliliters
1 tablespoon = ½ fluid ounce = 15 milliliters
2 tablespoons = 1 fluid ounce = 30 milliliters
¼ cup = 2 fluid ounces = 60 milliliters
⅓ cup = 2⅔ fluid ounces = 79 milliliters
½ cup = 4 fluid ounces = 118 milliliters
1 cup or ½ pint = 8 fluid ounces = 250 milliliters
2 cups or 1 pint = 16 fluid ounces = 500 milliliters
4 cups or 1 quart = 32 fluid ounces = 1,000 milliliters
1 gallon = 4 liters

Volume (Dry) Measurements

¼ teaspoon = 1 milliliter
½ teaspoon = 2 milliliters
¾ teaspoon = 4 milliliters
1 teaspoon = 5 milliliters
1 tablespoon = 15 milliliters
¼ cup = 59 milliliters
⅓ cup = 79 milliliters
½ cup = 118 milliliters
⅔ cup = 158 milliliters
¾ cup = 177 milliliters
1 cup = 225 milliliters
4 cups or 1 quart = 1 liter
½ gallon = 2 liters
1 gallon = 4 liters

Linear Measurements

½ in = 1½ cm
1 inch = 2½ cm
6 inches = 15 cm
8 inches = 20 cm
10 inches = 25 cm
12 inches = 30 cm
20 inches = 50 cm

Oven Temperature Equivalents, Fahrenheit (F) and Celsius (C)

100°F = 38°C	350°F = 180°C
200°F = 95°C	400°F = 205°C
250°F = 120°C	450°F = 230°C
300°F = 150°C	

Weight (Mass) Measurements

1 ounce = 30 grams
2 ounces = 55 grams
3 ounces = 85 grams
4 ounces = ¼ pound = 125 grams
8 ounces = ½ pound = 240 grams
12 ounces = ¾ pound = 375 grams
16 ounces = 1 pound = 454 grams